MW00574941

To my Dad:
Master gardener of
kindness, creativity, and joy

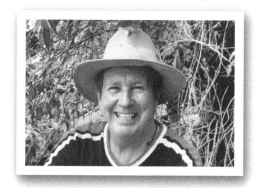

Paperback ISBN: 978-1-63732-213-0

COPYRIGHT: © 2021 Erin Fletter Books LLC
All Rights Reserved

All rights reserved. No part of this publication may be reproduced,
distributed, or transmitted in any form or by any means, including
photocopying, recording, or other electronic or mechanical methods,
without the prior written permission of the publisher, except in the
case of brief quotations embodied in critical reviews and certain other
noncommercial uses permitted by copyright law. For permission requests,
contact Erin Fletter at: https://stickyfingerscooking.com/contact

Cover and book design by Joe Hall.

FROM THE

Sticky Fingers Cooking™

SCHOOL

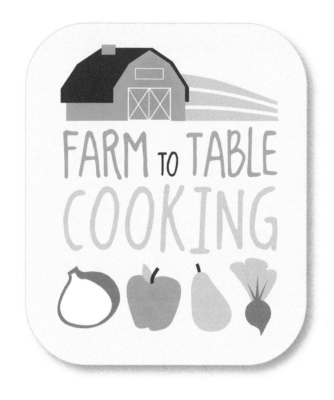

The Second Cookbook

FARM TO TABLE

"Wow, this is really crazy good stuff I just made..!"
-Young Chef Jason, age 7

"I HAVE to tell my mom about this recipe because I never eat vegetables and, wow, I love this!!"
-Young Chef Jordan, age 7

"This is so awesome; I love it!"
-Young Chef Haven, age 11

the STICKY FINGERS COOKING school ™

Sticky Fingers Cooking is an acclaimed mobile and online children's cooking school providing inspiring "hands-on" cooking classes to over 50,000 students since 2011. We recognize the value of fostering curiosity, independence, confidence, and development of essential, lifelong cooking skills through interactive and engaging culinary experiences.

We whisk together a sense of fun within all of our specially-developed, kid-friendly curriculum and in our over 800 proprietary recipes designed to expand children's skills and palates. We combine and connect our love of culinary arts with nutritional information, safe cooking skills, language, geography, math, science, and food history to help inspire and ignite a lifetime love of healthy cooking and adventurous eating that children relish.

"These are so delicious! I'm never going to stop eating them!!"
-Young Chef Ava, 2nd grade

"My parents aren't going to believe I made this! It's so good! I LOVE COOKING!!"
-Young Chef Grayson, age 8

"Sometimes, I think when I eat healthy food it tastes better than regular food."
-Young Chef Daniel, age 7

"I am constantly inspired by how all the young chefs in our cooking classes always love discovering the joys of fresh new flavors!"
- Erin Fletter

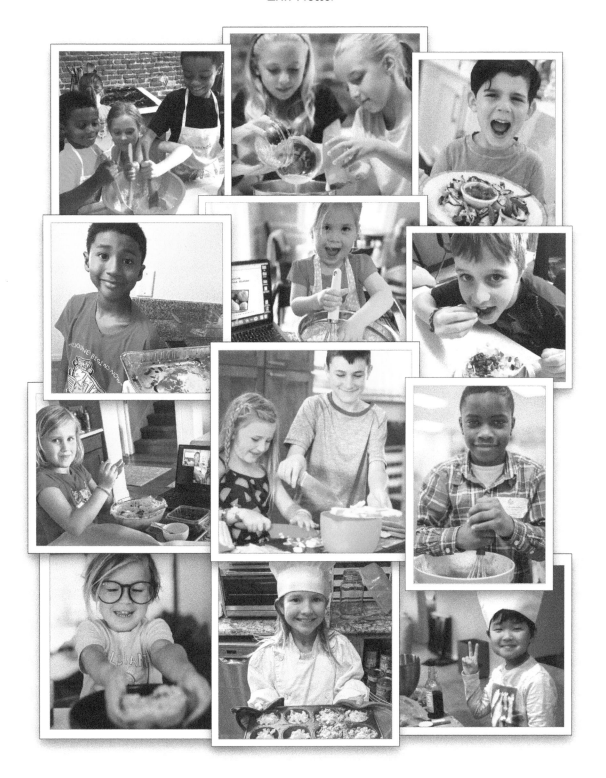

"I love everything we cook with Sticky Fingers!"
-Young Chef Gideon

People move
off farms,
the connection
to their local food
sources is
reduced.

Rachel Carson
publishes best
selling 'Silent Spring'
highlighting the
many dangers of
pesticides.

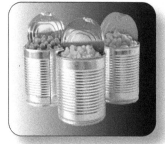
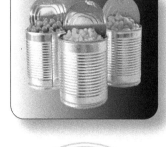

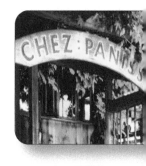

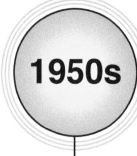

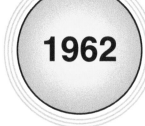

1940s

1950s

1962

1971

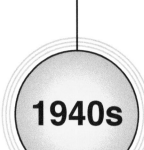
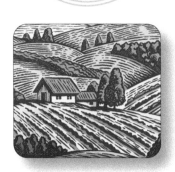

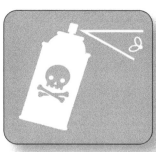

Packaged foods
explode with
innovations in food
processing and
storage, like cans
and frozen dinners.

Alice Waters, a
pioneering
advocate of
local, sustainable
agricure, opens
the ground breaking
legendary
Chez Panisse.

Carlo Perini, concerned about the quality-of-life impacts of fast food, founds the Slow Food Organization in Italy.

School learning gardens multiply, inspired by Alice Waters' Edible Schoolyard Project, as students learn all about loving to grow and eat fresh, healthy food.

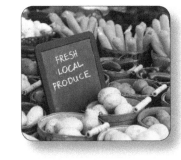

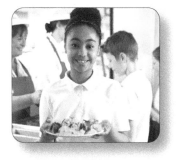

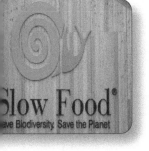

1986

1990s

2000s

2010s

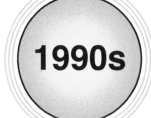

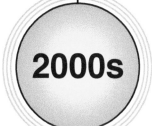

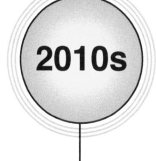

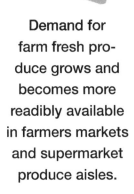

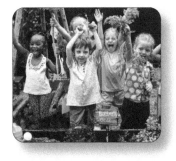

Demand for farm fresh produce grows and becomes more readibly available in farmers markets and supermarket produce aisles.

More and more schools start adding fresh, healthy, local foods to thier lunch program.

7

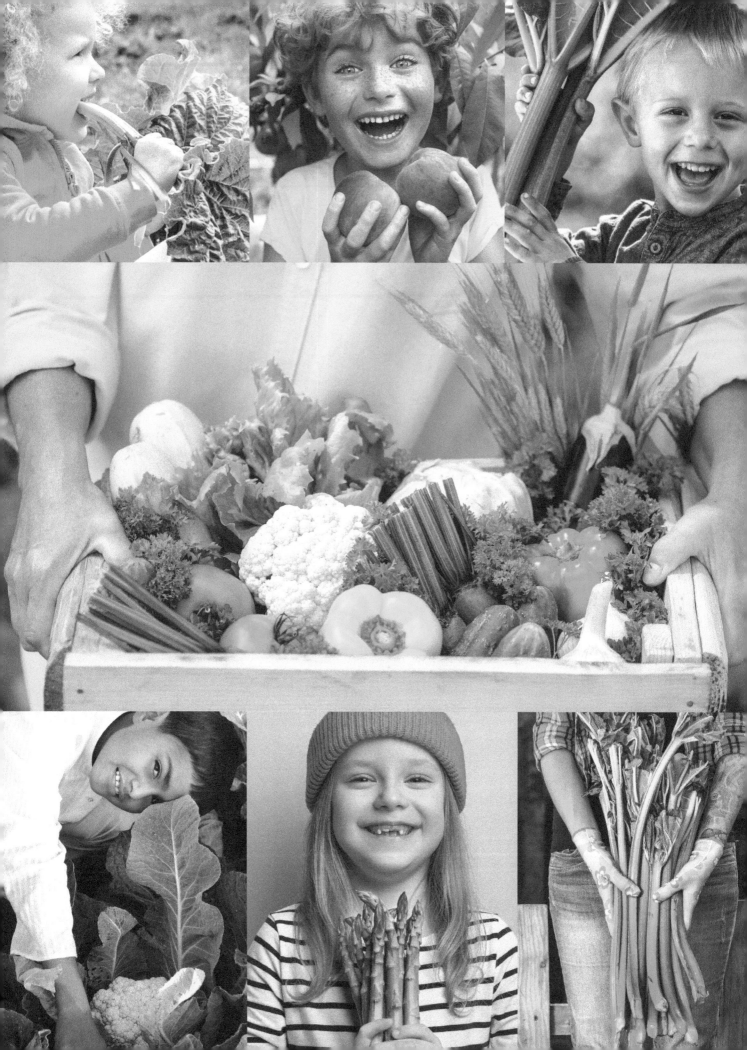

SPRING

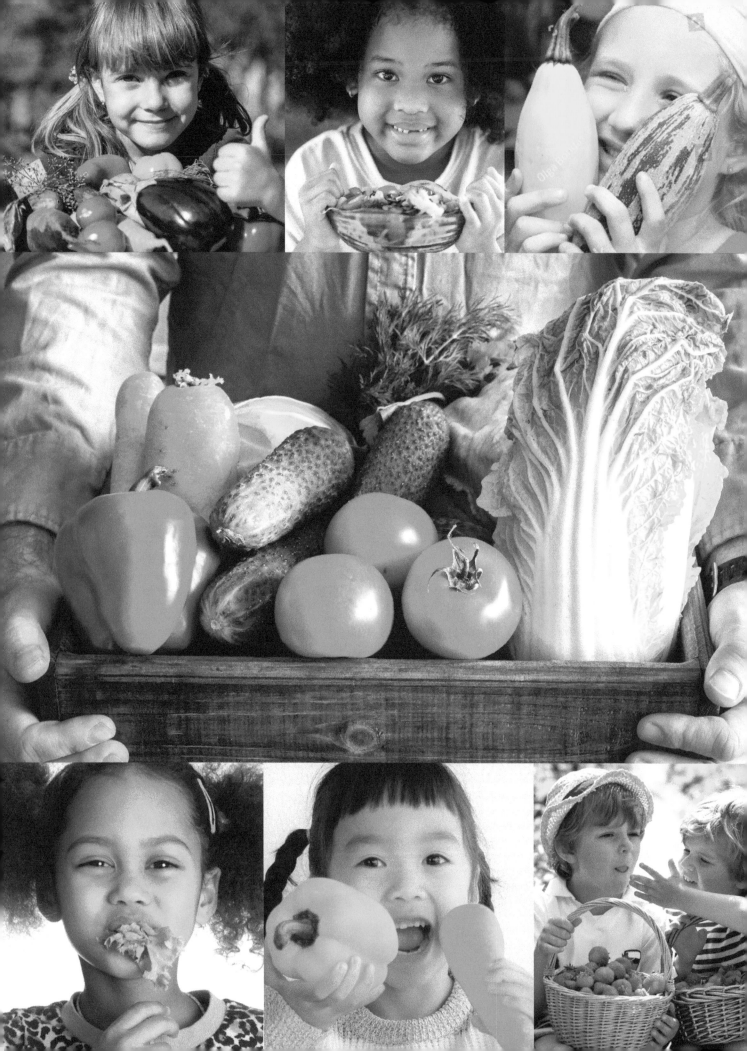

SUMMER

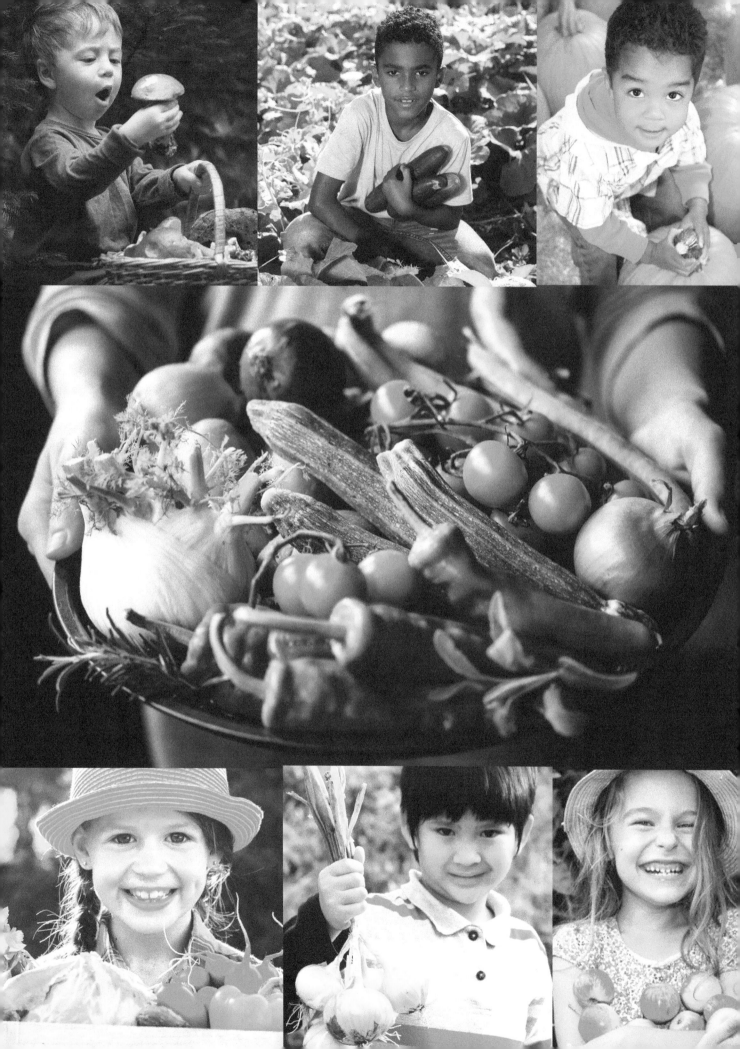

FALL

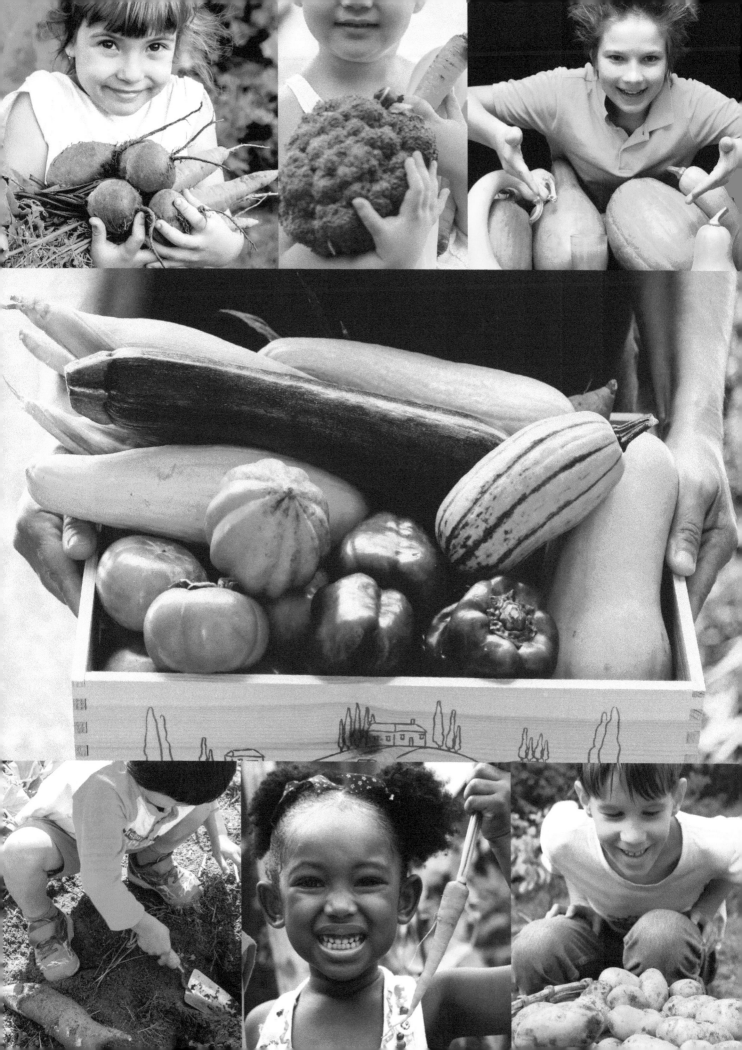

WINTER

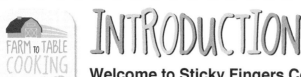

INTRODUCTION

Welcome to Sticky Fingers Cooking's Farm to Table Cookbook!

To me, the phrase "Farm to Table" means exploring new vegetables, planting gardens, going to a farmers market, visiting a farm, or even exploring the grocery store produce section to choose foods that you've never had before. It's about being thankful, it's about love, and it's about connection to people and our earth.

Growing up I was always an adventurous, robust, and passionate eater, but I never cooked all that much. Motherhood catapulted me into cooking. Living in a three-story, Victorian walk-up in San Francisco with a new baby, I found necessity and art colliding. I walked to neighborhood farmers markets to get inspiration and find the freshest produce that I could. I would talk to the local farmers. I would often decide right then and there what I would prepare for dinner each evening. I was hooked. Buying fresh, local produce and then cooking it became a way for me to express my creative side, and it became my ultimate expression of my love to my family. To me, to feed people well is to tell them you love them.

My husband Ryan and I went on to raise three beautiful kids in Colorado. At our local farmers market, our kids discovered — and could not stop eating — baby purple artichokes, something we would never have found at our local grocery store. We went back as often as we could to buy more for our dinner and to thank our local farmer.

Did you know that kids who regularly eat meals with their parents tend to eat more fruits and vegetables and are more likely to be physically and emotionally healthy? The benefits of planned family meals go way beyond nutrition, giving kids a balanced routine that creates stability and connectivity in their daily lives, and family mealtime conversations have been tied to improved literacy. Those occasions — like in our family, we have our special Fletter Family Fondue recipe that we only prepare and enjoy together on Christmas Eve — become important family bonding and memories, just as meaningful as any vacation or night out.

Food = Connection! Dinnertime is a wonderful time to be together after a busy day, and we like to make it a "special occasion." Yes, every dinner can be a special occasion. Being mindful of where food comes from, taking things slowly, appreciating and savoring. I was raised in a family where we all came together for dinner at the table, whether we were eating take-out pizza or making a nice dinner. And we maintain this habit still. We light candles, set the table, and come together to eat. Sometimes it's 15 minutes; sometimes it's three hours. But it's a daily ritual, and we are honoring our food and our time together.

The goal of farming is not just growing crops, but cultivating healthy human beings. The same rings true for cooking. Food brings people together in a way nothing else ever could. I am so thankful and awed by the connections that fresh food has brought to my life.

- Erin Fletter, Food-Geek-In-Chief, Co-Founder Sticky Fingers Cooking

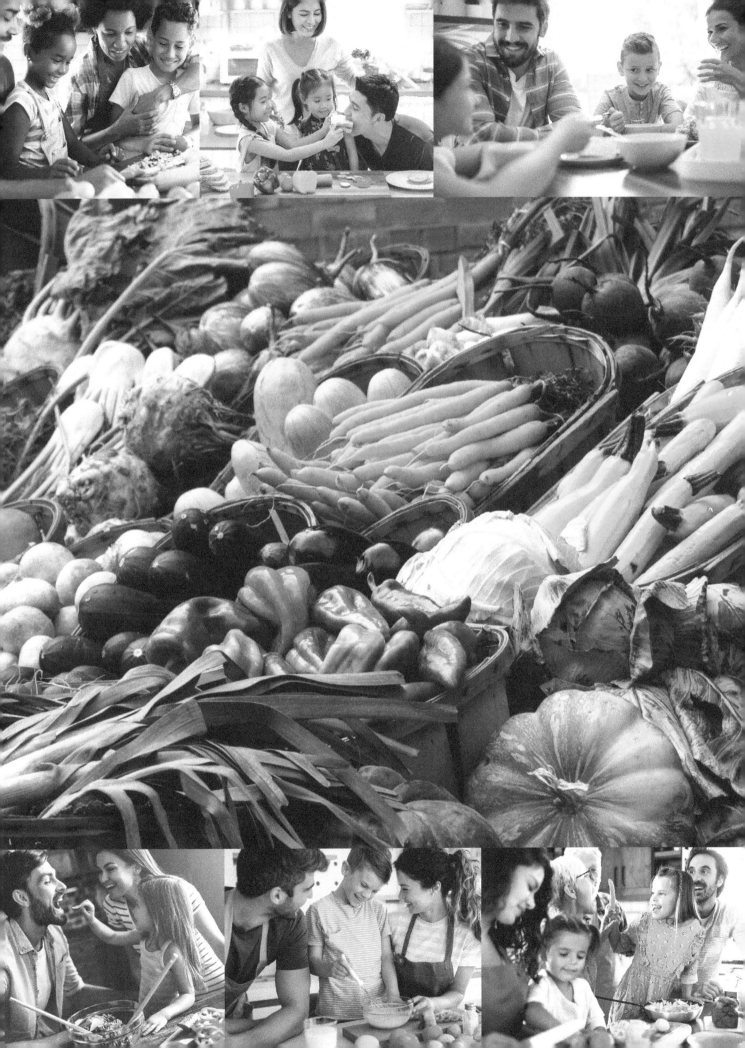

HOW TO USE THE COOKBOOK

In this scrumptious and inviting cookbook, young chefs and their families can cook 20 full-meal recipes that encourage the exploration and appreciation of new fruits and vegetables. You and your young chefs will prepare and savor flavorful, family-friendly cuisine inspired by seasonal, farm-fresh foods.

Cooking with kids is the most fun because it allows for creativity and flexibility. The motto we live by is "if they make it, they want to eat it." When kids take ownership of what they prepare and have a say in the recipe, they are more likely to try new foods and dishes. That is one of the driving forces behind the recipes crafted for this cookbook. The other is to make cooking colorful. When kids can see the rainbow on their plate, something magical happens; their eyes light up, and their natural curiosity and excitement are ignited.

Focusing on the beautiful food that nature creates for us is one of the best things about cooking. There's a mindfulness that comes with slowing down and appreciating the ingredients, the cooking process, the colors, the tastes. As you read through this book, you will notice our recipes highlight the magic that comes from using fresh, seasonal ingredients in your cooking.

You'll also notice these recipes are much more than stand-alone recipes. We encourage you and your kids to explore different pairings … have fun mixing and matching! While our recipes do not include many, if any, meat products, that's not to say you couldn't add your favorite proteins. We encourage you to find ways to make these recipes your own. The most important recipes are those that are most relevant to you and your family. Be bold and colorful in the kitchen!

In addition to the recipes, you will find invitations to connect with food and each other through kid-friendly activities, fun facts, and — of course — corny jokes! Kids can continue to improve on their skills as budding chefs by learning industry terminology and "how to" cooking techniques. You and your kids will be proud of all they can learn and accomplish.

After having taught over 55,000 (and counting) students in our cooking classes, seeing all the insanely creative kid creations is still the best part about what we do. We pride ourselves on our kid-tasted-and-approved content, and we are thrilled to offer this cookbook to you. We want your family to experience the joy of cooking and eating with people you love most.

We wish you happy and healthy cooking, always!

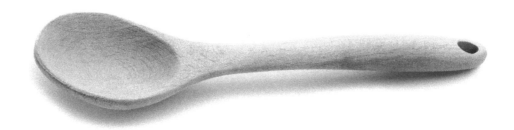

K'NIFTY KNIFE SKILLS

Why should you never argue with a knife? Because it will always have a good point!

We are getting straight to the point … get it? All jokes aside, we understand how intimidating handling kitchen blades can be (and how nerve-racking it can be for parents to watch!). Safety always comes first for us, and that is why we encourage you to use small, plastic lettuce knives, at least until you feel more confident and comfortable with your knife skills. The "teeth" of the knives are durable enough to cut through foods but not sharp enough to cause injury.

That being said, even with kid-friendly knives, accidents can still happen!

So, here a few tried-and-true reminders on handling knives in the kitchen:

DUH!: This may sound obvious, but take notice of which side is dull and which is sharp.

BE AWARE: Always walk with the knife tip down, and when you are finished using your knife, place it somewhere safe or in the sink.

MASTERY: For the best control, place your hand at the top of the handle where the blade and handle meet.

STABLE TABLE: Work on a stable, flat surface such as a cutting mat or board. Clear away items that might get in the way of you handling the knife.

LAY DOWN FLAT: Place any food flat-side down before cutting. It may be helpful for your parents to pre-cut food into pieces with flat surfaces, making it easier and safer for you to practice your skills!

HELP, PLEASE: Don't be afraid to ask an adult for help! We all need help sometimes, and asking for assistance can make the process go faster and be safer.

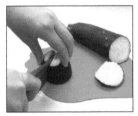

BRIDGE + TUNNEL (ZOOM, ZOOM!):
Place your non-knife hand above the food, holding the food in place between your fingers and thumb. The knife then goes underneath the "bridge" and into the "tunnel" so your hand is completely safe and cannot be cut. Saw back and forth.

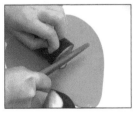

THE BEAR CLAW (GROWL!):
Curl all the fingers and the thumb of your non-knife hand like you're imitating a bear growling. Press the tips of your fingers (nails) to grip against the food, then saw back and forth.

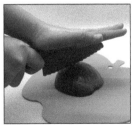

PLANK (SAW, SAW, SPLAT!):
Gently saw back and forth to make an initial cut in the food. Then, place your non-knife hand on top of the dull part of the knife to push down, adding extra pressure to cut through the food. Saw, saw, SPLAT!

SAW:
Practice making a sawing motion, "back and forth … back and forth."

CLEANING UP TIPS and TRICKS FOR KIDS

Just like how sports or board games follow rules to play, kitchens in restaurants have their own set of guidelines for safety and hygiene.

You will become an even more confident chef in the kitchen when you understand and master the following tips:

(A) **Always** Ask an Adult!

(B) **Beware** of Burners + Blades

(C) **Clean** your Clappers

(D) **Do** it as a Team

(E) **Eat & Enjoy Everything** (don't yuck my yum!)

(F) **FUN** is #1!

We can admit cleaning up is no one's favorite part about cooking. But imagine what the kitchen would look like (or smell like, ew) if we never cleaned after cooking — yikes! Cleaning, like anything else, though, can be more fun with laughter.

Try following these tips for keeping the kitchen clean and just remember to LAUGH:

(L) **Leave** a damp cloth nearby to wipe up messes or spills!

(A) **Ask** an adult which cleaning products should be used!

(U) **Use** prep stations to help keep you organized!

(G) **Get** rid of messes as you go!

(H) **Have** a garbage can close by to easily throw away scraps or trash!

Now that we've reviewed how to stay safe and clean in the kitchen, we are ready to get cooking! The best advice we can give for a fun and successful cooking experience is to **GO 1-2-3-SLOW** — that means do your best to prepare ahead of time so you don't have to worry while you're cooking. Like the story of the Tortoise and the Hare, slow and steady wins the race!

(1) **Always start by reading the recipe from top to bottom,** and then gather all of your ingredients and equipment for easy access.

(2) **For even easier prep, measure out all of your ingredients into small bowls ahead of time;** that way, when you go to use an ingredient, it is all ready and waiting for you!

(3) **Keep the cookbook open to your recipe in case you have to check back** or print the recipe off your tablet or device beforehand.

Remember, cooking is a process! We know it can be tempting to jump right into the actual cooking part, but taking the time to prepare will ensure a happier time in the kitchen. Think of it like going on vacation; it takes time to plan and prepare for all that fun!

CLEANING UP TIPS and TRICKS FOR PARENTS

"Our kitchen is clean enough to be healthy and messy enough to be happy."

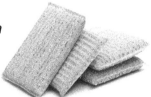

"Cleaning the kitchen is a spectator sport. My family watches me do it for hours."

Let's face it: cleaning is no one's favorite part about cooking, kids and parents included! We completely understand the struggles of getting kids to clean — we've all been there! The thing to keep in mind about cleaning, though, is it does not have to be perfect. The act of cleaning is just as important, if not more, than the result. We have a saying at Sticky Fingers Cooking: practice makes better, not perfect.

For toddlers, the physical movement that goes into cleaning helps develop their fine and gross motor skills. Think of some common cleaning responsibilities: twisting a lid closed on a jar, wiping down a dirty table, bringing dirty dishes to the sink. To adults, these tasks are automatic, but to developing children, they require a lot of communication and coordination between the brain and body!

For school-age children, the lesson of responsibility and the sense of accomplishment behind cleaning, whether or not kids appreciate it in the moment, make it a reward in and of itself. In fact, not feeling that sense of instant gratification from cleaning can lead to kids being able to handle frustration and adversity better later in life.

As you and your family clean up after your next meal, keep these tips in mind:

★ **Cleaning is not a punishment!** It's simply a part of life, just like brushing your teeth or washing your hands.

★ **Clean as a team!** If you all work together, no one feels singled out, and kids can feel the camaraderie that comes with working as a team.

★ **Make it a game!** Set a timer for, say, ten minutes and see who can clean the most within that time.

★ **Keep it bite-sized!** Focusing only on a couple tasks makes the job seem much more manageable to kids.

★ **Be flexible!** Keep in mind your kids probably won't be able to clean as well as you, and that's okay.

★ **Play your kids' favorite music!** Dancing while you work is always a fun time.

What's the most important part about cooking and cleaning? The time spent with each other. However you decide to approach the aftermath of cooking, find what works for you and your family.

EAT THE RAINBOW

Nutrition is a complex word. The truth is ... there is no one way to get the nutrition our bodies need, and different bodies need different nutrition! So how do you teach this to a 7-year-old?

Here's a simple trick: try to eat your way through the colors of the rainbow. We teach kids to eat as many different colors as they can. And no, we don't mean Skittles!

The colors represented in the fruits and vegetables we eat suggest their nutritional benefits. For example, you might have heard that carrots are good for your eyesight, and that's true! Carrots contain the pigment beta carotene that not only gives carrots their orange-yellow color but helps your body absorb vitamin A, which — you guessed it — is good for your eyes!

Try preparing a plate of options with just one or two colors represented. Perhaps for red, slice up a red bell pepper, tomato, and watermelon; for green, cut up a green bell pepper, broccoli, and cucumber. Let your kid choose what they want to eat from the plated options! Having choice can make kids feel more brave and empowered.

GREEN	WHITE	YELLOW
Helps keep you from catching a cold! leafy greens are loaded with vitamin C, which helps the body fight off invading germs.	Gives you energy! the natural sugars and carbohydrates in foods like potatoes, mushrooms, and cauliflower give your body a boost.	Helps make your bones strong! lemons and butternut squash contain vitamin A, which helps the body heal hurt tissue and grow strong bones and teeth.

ORANGE	BLUE/PURPLE	RED
Good for your heart! oranges and nectarines have lots of potassium, which helps your heart stay healthy so it can pump blood throughout your body.	Good for your brain! blueberries and eggplant have flavonoids that can improve memory and lots of antioxidants that rid the body of toxins.	Good for your blood! strawberries, beets, and red peppers have antioxidants that help red blood cells stay healthy.

Now, we know what you're thinking. All of this sounds great in theory, but how do I actually get my kid to eat green-colored foods?! We get it, and honestly not all colors of the rainbow will appeal to every kid's appetite. This is where a bit of creativity and flexibility can come into play: try making a fun rainbow chart together, and every time your kid eats a color of the rainbow, they can check it off! Taking ownership of what they are eating can help them overcome the picky-eater syndrome.

SPRING

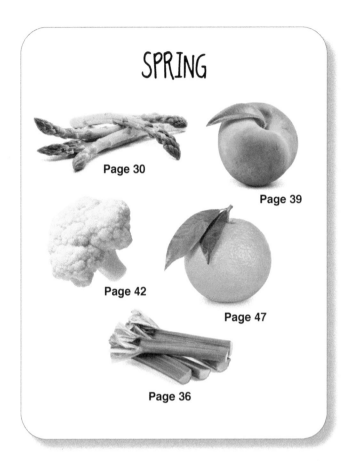

Page 30

Page 39

Page 42

Page 47

Page 36

SUMMER

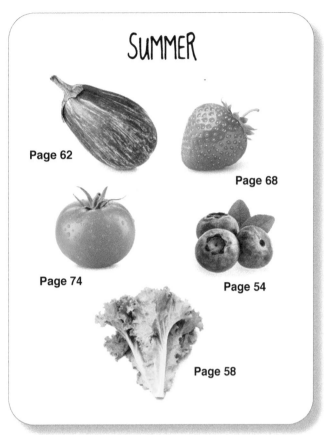

Page 62

Page 68

Page 74

Page 54

Page 58

FALL

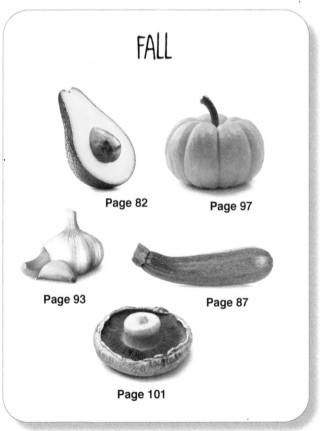

Page 82

Page 97

Page 93

Page 87

Page 101

WINTER

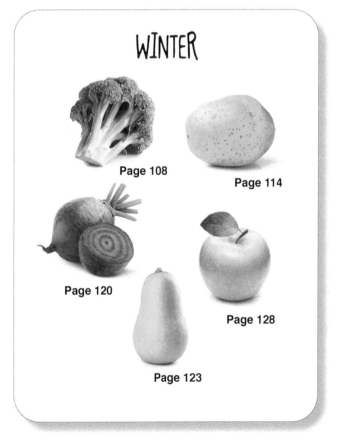

Page 108

Page 114

Page 120

Page 128

Page 123

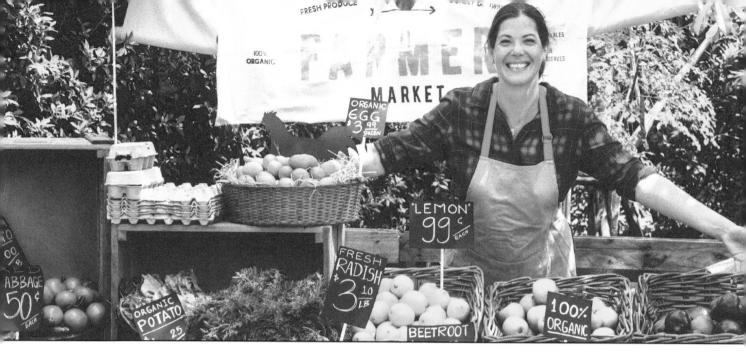

EAT LOCAL, SUPPORT LOCAL

Farmers selling their produce at local markets is an age-old tradition, yet as grocery stores grew in number, farmers markets began to fade into the background. In the last 50 years or so, however, farmers markets have made a big comeback, and with good reason!

There's nothing quite like eating produce from your local farmers market! Produce that comes directly from the farm with minimal processing is guaranteed to give you and your family not only the best taste but the most nutrition as well. Produce is fresher, brighter, and crisper when it only has to travel from the farm to the market, rather than making multiple stops in shipping on the way to the grocery store. You can feel good about knowing where your fruits and vegetables come from considering it's all seasonal food.

Farmers markets also offer an experience that grocery stores, though still wonderful, cannot quite replicate. When you're wandering from stall to stall, the sights, smells, and sounds of the farmers market can excite people of all ages. Picture produce of all shapes, sizes, and colors, or imagine the sizzle of corn on the cob blistering on a charcoal grill … Have you ever seen hatch chile peppers being roasted in a tumbler? It's a sight to behold, and a delicious aroma your nose won't soon forget! All five senses are sure to be enriched with a simple stroll through the market.

Visiting your local farmers market gives you another opportunity that your grocery store can't — the chance to speak with the farmers who grow your food! You can learn more about how and where the food is produced, and getting to know your local farmer can foster a sense of community. Farmers directly benefit from your support, so we call this a WIN-WIN!

Opportunities for experiences like these can make a lasting impression on kids, whether you visit your local farmers market regularly or just once. For more fun at the market, check out our Farmers Market Family Scavenger Hunt on page 51!

GATHERING AT THE DINNER TABLE

We know gathering for meals as a family can be a challenge. One kid has piano lessons, another has basketball practice, and somewhere in between schooltime and bedtime, homework has to happen. However, studies show that gathering for meals at the table can have a lasting, positive effect on kids. Kids thrive on routine, and carving out that time, whether it's ten minutes or an hour, to gather for a meal becomes something kids look forward to; it's time to decompress from the pressures of the day and enjoy nourishment for heart, mind, body, and soul — for you and your kids!

We have two secrets for making it to the table together:

1. **It doesn't have to be every day!** Try setting aside one or two days a week to purposefully gather. Once it becomes part of your routine, it's easier to gather more frequently.

2. **It doesn't have to be for dinner!** Maybe breakfast time works better for your family's schedule, or brunch on the weekends. It doesn't matter when you're eating, just that you're eating together.

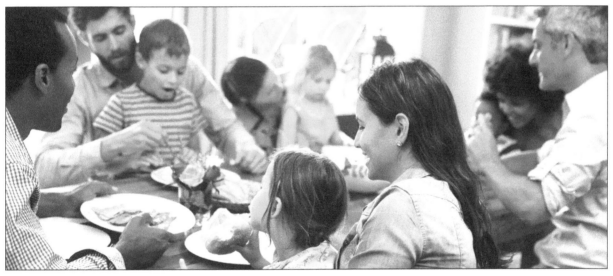

Also, there's something to be said for quality time spent together. Conversations and active participation at the table can go a long way in your kid's overall wellbeing. Here are some tips for making your time together quality:

- **This might seem obvious and redundant, but put away the phones.** This goes for you, too, parents! Try designating a specific place for your family to put their phones during meal times so the temptation to check is removed.

- **Involve the whole family to help prepare.** Even little ones can help set the table or fold napkins, and when kids have a responsibility, they are proud of their contribution and accomplishment.

🚜 **Find unique ways to engage your kids in conversation.** Ever asked your kid how their day at school went and you receive nothing but crickets? It's a tale as old as time. But kids respond to fun, off-the-wall conversation starters like "Would you rather only eat spaghetti for the rest of your life or hotdogs?"

🚜 **Avoid looking at the clock.** This one is harder than it might seem but so worth it in the end. When you're checking the time constantly, thinking about errands you need to run or things you need to do, the quality of time spent together is diminished. Try scheduling your gathering time on days when you know you don't have any meetings or practices, so you can be fully present with your family, without that clock face looming over you.

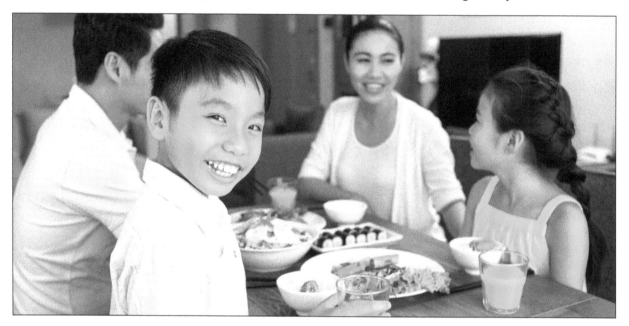

Table Setting Facts!

🚜 **In the Middle Ages, utensils at the table were not very common!** Other than a spoon for ladling soups or stews, most people ate with their fingers.

🚜 **Table cutlery was finally introduced in the 1600s** from people accidentally puncturing their mouths while using personal daggers to eat their food!

🚜 **Before the mid-1700s, most people ate "family style,"** much like we do today! Food was served on platters or in large bowls for people to share at the table.

🚜 **The seat next to the host was reserved for honored guests!**

🚜 **It was customary for gentlemen to stand when a woman or dignified dinner guest entered the room** and until they sat down at the table. This action was a symbol of respect.

🚜 **It was considered good manners to wait until everyone at the table was served before eating.** Also, etiquette called for cutting up only one or two bites of food at a time.

INVITING OUR IMAGINATION TO DINNER

- **Bring the outside in!** Using elements from nature is both fun and sustainable. Before dinner, try taking a field trip to the backyard or a nearby park to find inspiration for table decor. Perhaps you find an array of fallen pine cones to use for a fall feast, or maybe you snip fresh herbs or flowers from the garden for a springtime soiree!

- **Get crafty with your creations!** Making your table decor from scratch is a great activity for kids to explore their creativity and self-expression. Tip: Instead of recycling your empty bottles or cans, save them for future craft use!

- **Try DIY placemats!** Let your kids' imaginations run wild as they design placemats for everyone at the table. Construction paper, card stock, or felt make excellent placemats, and you could even laminate them yourself by sandwiching the placemats between two sheets of self-adhesive contact paper.

- **Go crayon crazy!** Using a large roll of brown craft paper, completely cover the table with paper and lay crayons or markers around the table to doodle while you eat! Tip: Check the thickness of your paper if using markers to ensure nothing bleeds through onto your table surface.

- **Set the mood!** We love this dinnertime ritual because it takes almost no time at all but can become a fun family tradition. Light a candle or two at the dinner table and play background music. Perhaps a different family member chooses the music each dinner!

- **Fold napkins in a fun way!** Search for napkin folding tutorials on the Internet to elevate your napkin game. Following procedural steps can provide mental stimulation for children, and the act of folding napkins lets little hands practice fine motor skills. Tip: Square, cloth napkins are more durable than paper and less frustrating or fiddly for kids. Plus, they can be used over and over again!

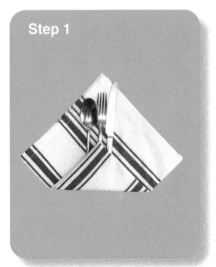
Step 1

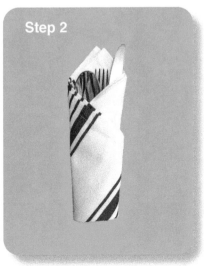
Step 2

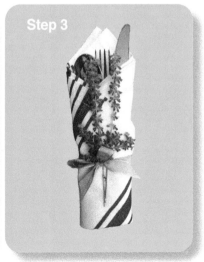
Step 3

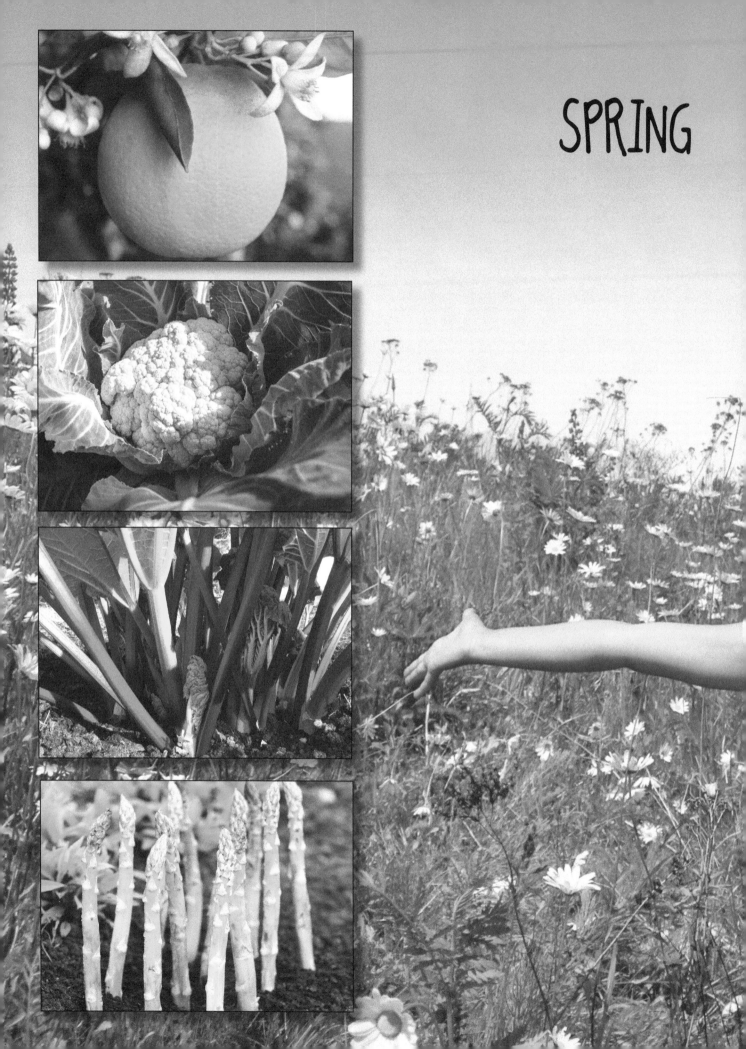

Why, hello there, Spring! Nothing tastes better than the first few meals in the Spring—light, bright, and bursting with freshly grown flavors. Sour rhubarb, crisp asparagus, tender peaches, crunchy cauliflower, and vivid citrus fruits are some of our favorite farm-fresh produce to celebrate this beautiful, unfolding new season!

"To plant a garden is to believe in tomorrow." - *Audrey Hepburn*

"Spring is nature's way of saying 'Let's Party!'" - *Robin Williams*

Laugh Time: How excited do farmers get about springtime? So excited they wet their plants.

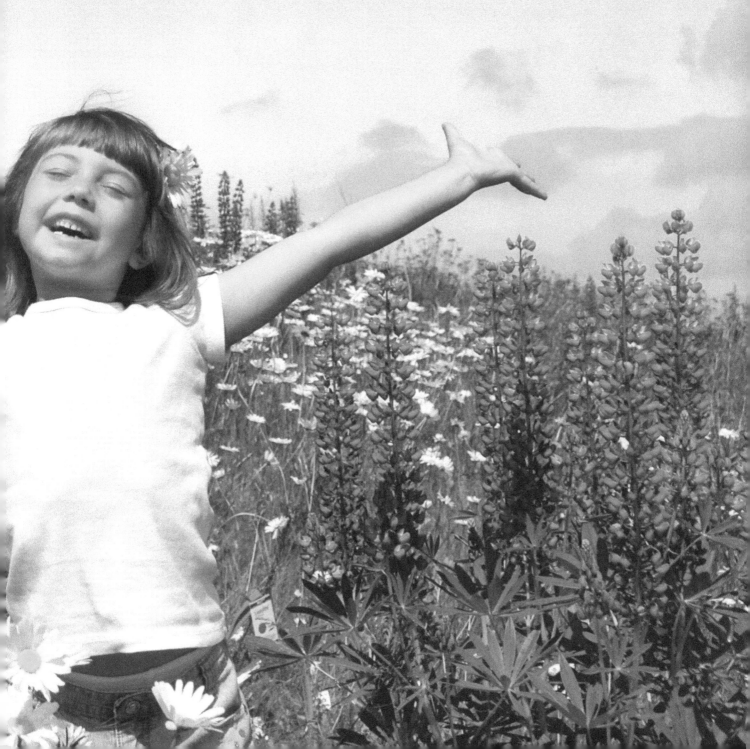

Spring Green Asparagus Ramen Bowl + Frizzled Spring Onions + Japanese Melon Coolers

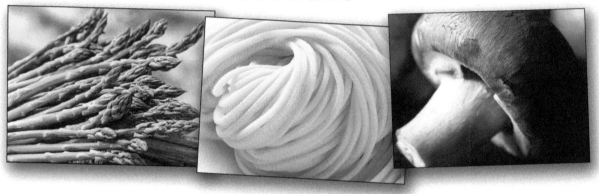

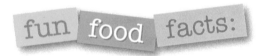

The History of Ramen

Ramen has a surprising origin; though it is considered a traditional Japanese dish, ramen was actually created by Chinese cooks in a restaurant in Tokyo in the early 1900s. They paired broth with Chinese noodles, which were more elastic and yellower in color compared to Japanese noodles. At that point, the dish was called *shina soba*, based on the phonetic word for "China."

About 50 years later, the instant ramen noodle that we know today was invented. The convenience of cooking noodles in a cup became wildly appealing, and why wouldn't it? People could easily enjoy ramen noodles away from the home, in school or at work. As instant ramen noodles became more mainstream in the market, the hunger to improve upon its flavor helped this delicious dish evolve.

Japan is home to an impressive 35,000 ramen noodle restaurants today, each one taking pride in its own, special recipe.

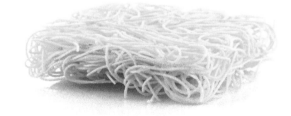

The featured ingredient: Asparagus!

★ **Asparagus comes from a perennial plant,** meaning asparagus shoots will return every year once the plant is established. They are one of the first plants to greet us in the spring-time because their roots can grow up to 6 inches of edible spears in only 24 hours!

★ **Asparagus gets its name from the Greek word *asparagos*,** which is thought to mean "to spring up."

★ **The spears of an asparagus plant grow from an underground crown,** which is made up of fleshy roots called rhizomes. As the spears grow, they become glossy and tender, with many triangular bumps called bracts appearing toward the tops.

★ **Green isn't the only color of asparagus: it also comes in white and purple!** White asparagus grows completely underground, unlike green asparagus spears. Since they then lack the necessary sunlight to undergo photosynthesis (a process that gives plants a green color), they stay white!

★ **Asparagus has lots of vitamins including calcium, folate, vitamin E, and vitamin K, as well as dietary fiber.**

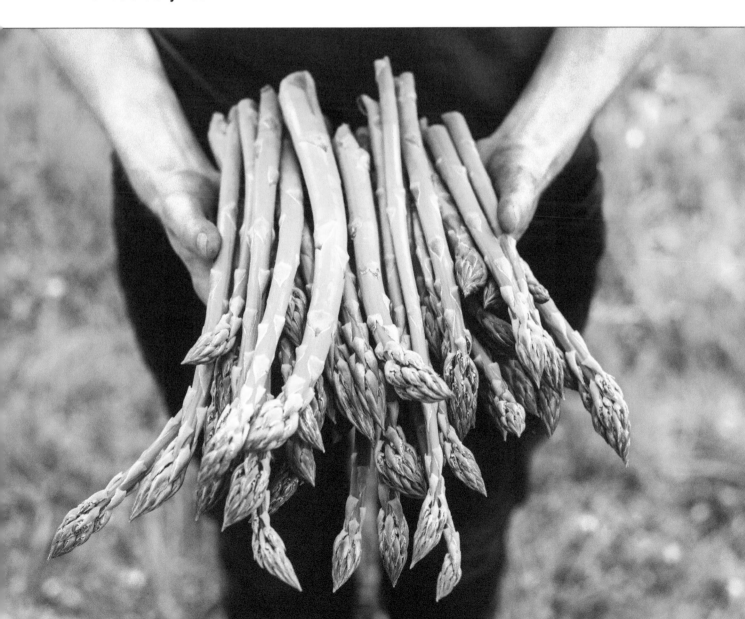

spring green asparagus ramen bowl

ingredients

8 to 10 asparagus spears, preferably thick stalks

8 to 10 mushrooms

1 smashed garlic clove

2 T miso paste (red, white or yellow)

½ tsp sugar or honey

½ tsp salt

2 two-inch squares kombu seaweed (or sub 1 sheet toasted nori seaweed or ¼ C wakame seaweed)

6 to 9 oz dried ramen noodles (or sub rice ramen noodles for GF)

optional toppings:

extra kombu, nori, or wakame seaweed

sliced radishes

handful bean sprouts

bamboo shoots

corn kernels

2 to 4 large hard-boiled eggs

drizzle sesame oil

drizzle soy sauce

splash rice wine vinegar

squeeze lemon or lime juice

snap+dice+slice

First make the Frizzled Spring Onions (see recipe on page 33). No need to clean out saucepan after removing onions before making the ramen!

Have kids snap off the tough ends of **8 to 10 asparagus spears** and snap off the stems of **8 to 10 mushrooms.** Save mushroom stems for broth and then dice up the asparagus tips and slice up the mushroom caps.

sauté+add+simmer

Sauté the mushroom stems and **1 smashed garlic clove** for 2 to 3 minutes in your saucepan on your stovetop over medium heat. Turn off the heat and add 5 cups of water, **2 tablespoons of miso paste, ½ teaspoon of sugar or honey, ½ teaspoon of salt, 2 two-inch squares of kombu.** Turn your saucepan back on high and bring to a boil. Reduce heat and simmer for 10 to 20 minutes.

strain+discard+adjust

Strain out and discard the mushroom stems, garlic, and seaweed from the saucepan with a slotted spoon. Taste the broth and adjust, adding more miso, salt and honey or sugar, if necessary.

add+cook+garnish

Add **6 to 9 oz of dried ramen noodles** (or rice noodles for gluten-free version) and cook until noodles are tender, about 4 to 7 minutes. Divide ramen among bowls to serve and then garnish with extra seaweed, or any other optional toppings, including **sliced radishes, bean sprouts, bamboo shoots, corn kernels, hard-boiled egg halves, drizzle of sesame oil, drizzle of soy sauce, splash of rice wine vinegar, or a squeeze of fresh lemon or lime.** Finally, garnish with *Frizzled Spring Onions!*

● ●

frizzled spring onions

ingredients

½ bunch green onions
4 T oil

salt to taste

trim+slice

Have your kids trim and slice **1/2 bunch of green onions** into 3-inch matchsticks.

heat+frizzle

Heat **4 tablespoons of oil** in a saucepan on your stovetop over medium heat. Test the temperature by adding a piece of green onion: it will sizzle on contact when the oil is hot enough. Add the green onions and cook, stirring frequently, until brown all over, but not burned.

transfer+sprinkle+cool

Use a slotted spoon or spatula to transfer the frizzled onions to a paper-towel-lined plate. Sprinkle with **salt** and allow to cool. Serve on top of ramen!

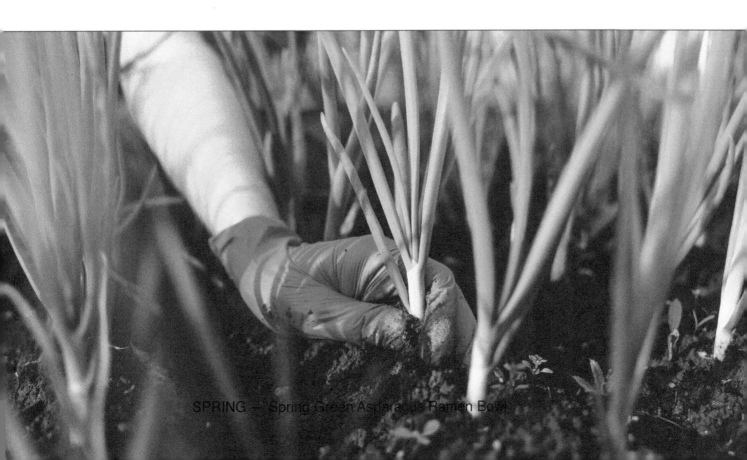

japanese melon coolers

ingredients

½ melon, either watermelon or cantaloupe

½ C sugar or honey

2 C ice

salt to taste

chop+blend

Have kids remove seeds and chop up ½ **melon, either watermelon or cantaloupe.** Add chopped melon, along with 1 cup of water, into your blender or a pitcher for use with a hand blender. Blend until smooth.

add+blend

Add ½ **cup of sugar or honey** and **2 cups of ice.** Add salt to taste. Blend again until smooth and thick.

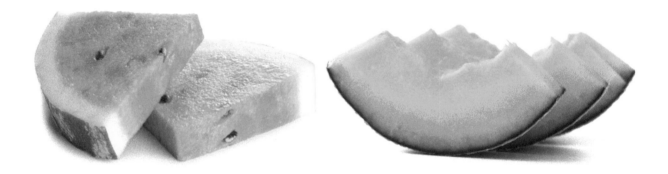

Time for a Laugh!

What did the asparagus say to the bowl of ramen soup?
Stop STALKING me!

How did the bowl of asparagus ramen soup reply?
But you make MISO happy!

thyme for a fun activity

From Scraps to Hacks!

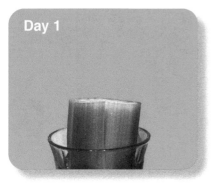

Day 1

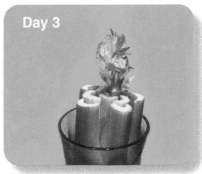

Day 3

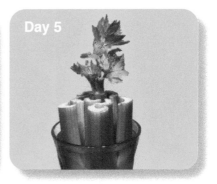

Day 5

🚜 **The simplest way to reuse old table scraps, such as the bottoms of bell peppers or the tops of turnips, is to compost them!** Place your leftover scraps in a dedicated compost bin or area, and let nature do its work. When organic materials decompose (or break down into smaller parts), they release nutrients that fertilize soil to help plants grow.

🚜 **The next time you eat a banana and go to throw away the peel, STOP!** Did you know that peel can help fertilize your plants? Chop the banana peel and add to a bowl, then fill the bowl with water. Let the peel soak in the water for a couple hours, but the longer, the better. As the banana peel soaks, it releases all of the nutrients, like manganese, potassium, calcium, and phosphorus. These are all things roots and stems need for healthy growth! Use this nutrient-dense water to quench your plant's thirst.

🚜 **When you have used up all the stalks of celery, save the bottom stem (the last inch or two) to regrow some more!** Place the stem (with the end where the stalks were cut pointing up) in a shallow bowl or glass filled with water, and then leave it in a sunny spot or on a windowsill. Change the water every 1-2 days, and soon you will see tiny new shoots springing up from where the stalks were cut! As the new stalks grow, you may need to peel off the old, outer layer as those will start to decay. When you start to see roots growing from the bottom of the stem, you know it's time to transplant your celery into soil and continue to let it grow.

🚜 **You can also regrow your green onions from the white bulbs that usually get thrown away. Save the last inch or so of your green onion stalks and place root down in ½ inch of water.** Make sure the water covers the roots but not the tops. Keep your green onion bulbs on the windowsill where it's easy to change the water, which you should do one to two times a week. You'll start seeing fresh shoots growing in a few days!

Wee Scottish Rhubarb Cream Cheese "Bridie" Hand Pies + Sticky Mandarin Glaze + Mandarin Orange Fizz

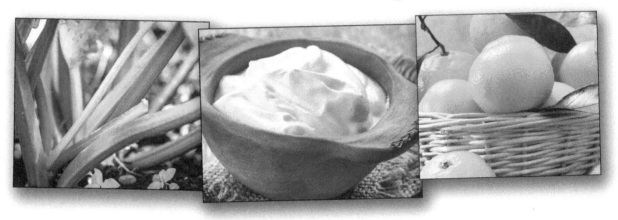

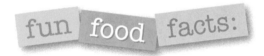

Let's Learn a Wee Bit About Rhubarb!

Rhubarb is native to China where it was used as medicine!

People began consuming rhubarb as food right around the same time that sugar became affordable and more widely available.

In the summertime in Alaska, rhubarb plants can grow over 5 feet tall! This is because of Alaska's long, sunny days during summer.

Rhubarb is a perennial plant. That means it'll come back year after year once planted (for at least 10 years).

The edible part of a rhubarb plant is the thick stalk (called petiole), which can vary in color from light green to deep red. Red rhubarb stalks are sweeter; green stalks are more sour. Rhubarb flesh is white.

FIBER! Rhubarb contains a healthy amount of fiber, which helps keep our intestines clean and running smoothly.

Let's Learn about Scotland!

Scotland is located in Europe at the northern end of Great Britain. Scotland is a part of the United Kingdom, along with England, Wales, and Northern Ireland.

Many species of wildlife can be found in Scotland, including seals, mountain hares, ptarmigans (similar to grouse), stoats (or weasels), and golden eagles.

The official animal of Scotland is the unicorn, loved for its purity and strength.

In Scotland, people drive ww**The thistle is a national symbol of Scotland.**

Scottish dishes are well known for their peculiar names, like Forfar Bridie (a meat pastry), Cock-a-leekie (soup), Collops (escalope), Crappit Heid (fish dish), Finnan Haddie (haddock fish), Arbroath Smokie (smoked haddock), Cullen Skink (haddock soup), Partan Bree (seafood dish), Mince and Tatties (minced meat and potatoes), Rumbledethumps (vegetable casserole), and Skirlie (savory oatmeal dish).

wee scottish rhubarb cream cheese "bridie" hand pies

ingredients

7 oz puff pastry (thawed)

½ C chopped rhubarb

¼ C sugar

1 tsp all-purpose flour

pinch salt

4 oz cream cheese, softened

defrost+chop+measure+mix

Overnight, defrost **7 oz puff pastry** in the fridge. When ready to bake, chop up ½ **heaping cup of rhubarb** into small pieces. Add to a mixing bowl. Measure and add ¼ **cup of sugar, 1 teaspoon of flour,** and **a pinch of salt** to the rhubarb. Mix! Then add **4 oz of cream cheese** and mix again. Let rhubarb rest for 30 minutes while you preheat your oven.

preheat+roll+cut

Preheat oven to 350 degrees F and line a baking sheet with parchment paper. Roll out puff pastry on a floured surface. Using the lid of a mason jar, cut out circular shapes in the puff pastry, making as many as you can, or cut out rectangles with a butter knife.

spoon+fold+seal+bake

Spoon 1 to 2 teaspoons of rhubarb cream cheese mixture in the center of each dough shape. Trace edges with a wet finger, then fold over and seal edges closed. Arrange on baking sheet, slide into the oven, and bake until puff pastry is golden brown and flaky and rhubarb filling is bubbly! Drizzle with *Sticky Mandarin Glaze* (recipe on page 38)!

sticky mandarin glaze

ingredients

¼ C powdered sugar

3 tsp mandarin juice (from 1 can mandarin oranges or 1 fresh mandarin/tangerine)

¼ tsp vanilla extract

pinch salt

measure+whisk+drizzle

Measure and whisk together ¼ **cup of powdered sugar, 3 teaspoons of mandarin orange juice** (or juice and zest from 1 fresh tangerine/mandarin), **¼ teaspoon of vanilla extract**, and **a pinch of salt.** Drizzle over baked *Bridie Hand Pies* and ENJOY!

mandarin orange fizz

ingredients

10.5 oz can mandarin oranges (or 3 fresh mandarins/tangerines)

1 C ice

2 C sparkling water

sugar to taste

add+puree+pour

Add a **10.5 oz can mandarin oranges** (or 3 freshly peeled tangerines/mandarins), **1 cup of ice, and 1 cup of sparkling water** to a blender. Puree until very smooth and thick, then add **1 more cup of sparkling water** and **sugar to taste.** Stir, pour, and drink up!

Let's Finish with a Laugh!

What water yields award-winning rhubarb? Perspiration!

Why was the rhubarb by himself? Because the banana split!

Why did the pie go to a dentist? Because he needed a filling!

Perfectly Peachy Panzanella Salad + Bellissima Basil Vinaigrette + Blended Basil Spring Peach-ade

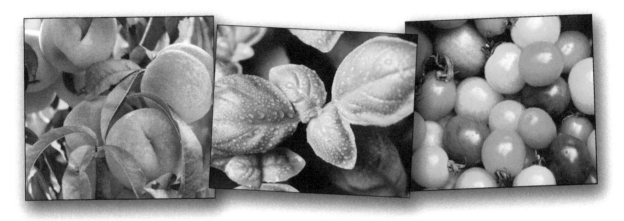

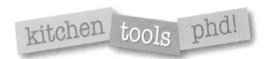

Slicing, Dicing, Mincing, Tearing, Whisking!

KITCHEN TOOLS PhD recipes help us get comfortable using common cooking tools in the kitchen, including our hands! Kitchen tools help young chefs develop and hone fine motor skills as they prepare savory, delicious recipes.

SLICE: to cut into pieces using a sawing motion with your knife.

DICE: to chop foods into small pieces of equal size so that the food is cooked evenly or looks uniform and pleasant when used in the recipe.

TEAR: to pull or rip something apart into pieces.

WHISK: to beat or stir with a light, rapid movement either with a fork or an appropriately named gadget called a whisk.

BLEND: to combine two or more ingredients together so that they lose their individual characteristics and become smooth and uniform.

A Brief History of Panzanella:

Panzanella (pahn-zah-NEHL-lah) was originally a Tuscan Italian recipe invented to make use of stale, day-old bread.

Bread used to be baked in communal ovens, so people would have to make the most of the bread they made for the entire week. They soaked the stale bread in water and vinegar and then mixed it with whatever fresh vegetables and tomatoes were available in the garden.

Until the 20th century, panzanella was a salad made with onions, not tomatoes.

Other ingredients added to panzanella include anchovies, lettuce, olives, mozzarella, white or red wine vinegar, celery, carrots, mint, boiled eggs, and capers. Peaches are certainly not traditional, but we're using them because they are SO good with summer tomatoes!

● ●

perfectly peachy panzanella salad + bellissima basil vinaigrette

ingredients

peachy panzanella salad ingredients:
2 C mixed cherry tomatoes
1 tsp sea salt (+ more to taste)
½ large baguette
2 T olive oil
pepper to taste
2 garlic cloves
2 ripe peaches
4 oz mozzarella cheese

bellissima basil vinaigrette:
¼ C red wine vinegar
¼ C olive oil
½ tsp sugar/honey/agave
handful fresh basil leaves

slice+sprinkle+drain

Slice **2 cups of mixed cherry tomatoes** into halves. Sprinkle with **1 teaspoon salt,** then put tomatoes in a colander set over a large mixing bowl. Let the tomatoes drain for about 30 minutes.

tear+toss+smash+toast

Tear ½ **a baguette** into rough 1-inch pieces and add them to a bowl. Add **2 tablespoons of olive oil** and **pinches of salt** and **pepper.** Toss to coat the bread with oil. Smash and peel **2 garlic cloves.** Toast bread cubes and smashed garlic in a dry skillet over medium heat. Once toasted, set aside the bread to cool and discard the garlic.

tear+dice+chop+whisk+toss

Tear a **handful of fresh basil leaves** into small bits. Dice **2 peaches** into small pieces. Chop **4 oz of mozzarella cheese.** Then whisk together ¼ **cup of red wine vinegar,** ¼ **cup of olive oil,** ½ **teaspoon of sugar/honey/agave,** and the torn basil leaves. Add this to a mixing bowl and toss the tomatoes and peaches with the dressing. Add the cheese and bread and toss gently again, then eat! Or as we say in Italian, *mangia bene!*

●●

blended basil peach-ade

ingredients

1 large ripe peach

2 large basil leaves (+ more for garnish)

2 to 4 lemons (for juicing)

½ C sugar

ice

dice+tear+squeeze

Dice **1 large ripe peach** into small pieces. Tear **2 basil leaves** and add them to a blender along with the diced peach. Squeeze juice from **2 to 4 lemons** into the blender.

measure+add+blend

Measure and add ½ **cup of sugar** and **2 cups of cold water** to your blender! Cover and blitz on high until drink is smooth and blended. Then pour the mixture over cups and add **ice** to chill. Garnish with basil leaves and enjoy!

Let's Finish with a Laugh!

How do you get rid of lazy tomato employees?
Can 'em!

Did you hear the joke about the peach?
It's pit-iful!

How do you make a peach into a vegetable?
Step on it and make it squash!

Totally Turkish Cauliflower Kofta Bites
+ Spiced Tomato Sauce + Herbaceous Haydari (Minted Yogurt Dip) + Sweet Blended Fresh Mint Tea

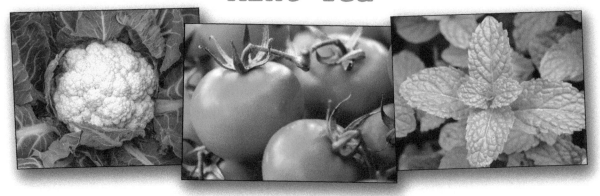

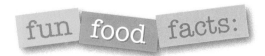

What is Kofta?

Kofta (KOFF-tah) is a member of the meatball family! Kofta are eaten all over the world, most commonly in the middle East, Southern Asia, or the Balkan areas. Traditionally, they are balls of minced or ground lamb, chicken, beef, or pork, and they are usually cooked on a grill or open flame.

The word *kofta* comes from the classical Persian verb *koftan*, which means "to pound" or "to grind," reflecting the ground meat used for the meatballs.

India serves versions of vegetarian kofta made from potato, calabash, paneer (cheese), and even banana, whereas fish and seafood kofta are commonly found in West Bengal, South India, Egypt, and parts of the Persian Gulf. In Albania, there are specialized shops called Qofteri offering kofta and beer. In Bulgaria, kofta consist of pork, veal, beef, or even a mixture of the three. In Iran and Pakistan, kofta are served with a spicy gravy while in Cypress and Greece

The featured ingredient: Mint!

★ **The mint herb dates back thousands of years.** Archeologists have found evidence of mint in Egyptian tombs dating back to 1000 BCE, and this fragrant herb has been a part of Chinese medicine for even longer.

★ **Romans used mint to scent their bathwater and perfume their bodies,** and some even wore wreaths of mint leaves around their heads or carried sprigs in their pockets. Not only did early Romans believe eating mint would increase intelligence, but they also thought the scent of mint could stop a person from losing their temper.

★ **Mint gets its name from Greek mythology!** Hades, the god of the underworld, fell in love with a river nymph name Minthe. When Hades' wife Persephone found out, she jealously turned Minthe into a plant so all could walk over and crush her. Hades was unable to undo Persephone's spell, so instead he gave Minthe a beautiful aroma to make up for her unfortunate situation.

★ **Peppermint is said to have a calming, cooling effect on the body, and it has been used as a home remedy to treat indigestion for years.**

★ **Mint comes in many varieties, more than 30!** Spearmint is the most common garden variety, but others include lavender mint, apple mint, licorice mint, and even chocolate mint!

★ **Mint is rich in vitamins A and C but also contains an antioxidant called rosmarinic acid known for its anti-inflammatory properties.**

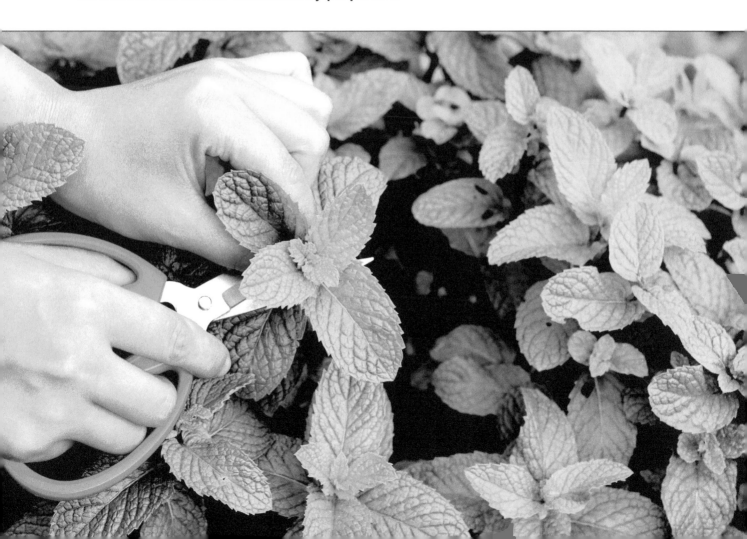

totally turkish cauliflower kofta bites

ingredients

1 pot water (boiling)
1 medium potato
1½ C cauliflower florets
2 green onions
1 garlic clove
½ C canned chickpeas (garbanzo beans), drained and rinsed

¼ tsp sugar or honey
pinch salt + black pepper
4 T vegetable oil
2 to 3 T all-purpose flour (as needed)
¼ tsp dried ground ginger, ground turmeric, ground cumin, ground coriander

boil+chop

First, bring a pot of water to boil, then add **1 medium potato** until it is cooked through (or you can use ¼ to ½ cup of pre-cooked, mashed potato instead). Remove from water and cool. Chop up **1½ cups of cauliflower florets, 2 green onions,** and **1 garlic clove** into tiny bits and set to side.

mash+measure

In a large bowl, mash together the boiled potato, ½ **cup of chickpeas** (garbanzo beans), ¼ **teaspoon of sugar or honey,** and **a pinch of salt** and **black pepper.** Then measure out ¼ **teaspoon each of ginger, turmeric, cumin,** and **coriander** into a small bowl.

heat+sauté

Meanwhile, heat **2 tablespoons of vegetable oil** in a skillet on your stovetop over medium heat. When hot, add the chopped cauliflower, garlic, and green onions, stirring until fragrant and soft, about 3 to 5 minutes. Add your spices and stir to coat. Transfer to a mixing bowl and set aside to let cool slightly.

combine+grind

Combine the chickpea/potato mixture with the cauliflower mixture. Then, using an immersion blender in the bowl or a food processor, grind the ingredients into a coarse paste.

form+fry

Form the mixture into small balls, adding a bit of **flour** to the mixture if the kofta don't come together and stick. Then, heat 1 to 2 tablespoons vegetable oil in a skillet on the stovetop and add the kofta, gently frying until golden brown all over. Remove and drain on paper towels while you make the *Spiced Tomato Sauce* (see recipe on page 45). Once the tomato sauce is finished simmering in your skillet, you will add the kofta back in to cover with sauce before serving!

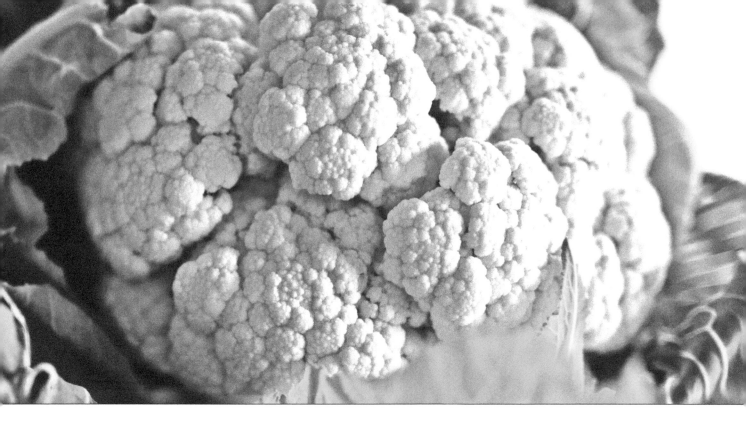

spiced tomato sauce

ingredients

½ garlic clove

2 tomatoes

pinch dried ginger

pinch ground turmeric

pinch ground cumin

pinch ground coriander

¼ tsp salt

squirt honey

1½ T vegetable oil

chop+pinch+squirt

Chop ½ **garlic clove** and **2 tomatoes** and combine in a bowl. Add **pinches of ginger, turmeric, cumin,** and **coriander** to the bowl, and then add ¼ **teaspoon of salt** and **a squirt of honey**, along with 1½ **tablespoons of vegetable oil.**

blend+simmer

Blend the ingredients up with an immersion blender in the bowl or pour into a blender or food processor. Then pour the sauce into your skillet on your stovetop and simmer for 3 to 5 minutes, covered, to cook and thicken.

combine+serve

Add the fried kofta back into your skillet and cover with the sauce prior to serving!

Optional: Serve kofta with sauce and yogurt dip with pita bread or corn tortillas.

herbaceous haydari

ingredients

½ garlic clove
3 fresh mint leaves
½ C full-fat Greek yogurt

big pinch salt
squirt honey

chop+tear+whisk

Chop ½ **garlic clove** and add to a small bowl. Tear up **3 mint leaves** and add to the bowl.

Measure and whisk in ½ **cup of full-fat Greek yogurt, a pinch of salt,** and **a squirt of honey.**

Spoon the yogurt dip over the kofta bites and enjoy!

sweet blended fresh mint tea

ingredients

7 fresh mint leaves
4 T sugar or honey

1 C ice

tear+blend+steep

Tear up **7 mint leaves** and add to a pitcher, along with 4 cups of warm water. Blend using an immersion blender or pour into blender. Let steep for at least 30 minutes.

add+blend

Add **4 tablespoons of sugar or honey** and **1 cup of ice** into the pitcher and blend together. ENJOY!

Let's Finish with a Laugh!

Knock-knock! Who's there? **Mint!** Mint, who?
I mint to ring the doorbell!

What did the kofta say to the minted yogurt dip?
We were mint for each other!

Springtime Citrus Cakelette Creations
+ Sweet-Tart Citrus Glazes
+ Citrus Peel Confetti Sprinkles
+ Easy Breezy Citrus-ade

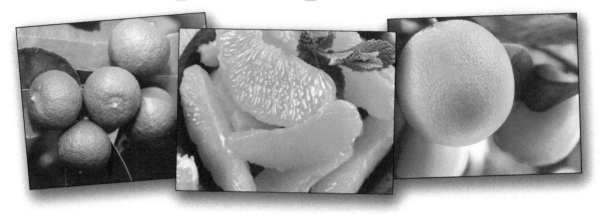

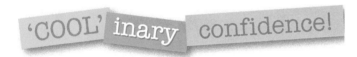

'COOL' inary confidence!

Slicing, Chopping, Mincing, Mixing, Blending!

SLICE: to cut into pieces using a sawing motion with your knife!

CHOP: to cut food into rough pieces that are not usually the same size!

MINCE: to cut food into teeny-tiny pieces!

What Can We Learn About Citrus?

Citrus fruits are a type of berry (surprise!) that have tough and leathery rinds, which are known as hesperidia. Out of the possible 60,000 flowers a single citrus plant can produce, only one percent of those flowers actually turn into a fruit.

Citrus plants originated in Southeast Asia. If they are grown in tropical climates without a proper winter, citrus fruits will maintain a green color on the outside.

Navel oranges get their name from the belly button-looking part on the bottom of the fruit!

Lemons were once so rare that they were presented to kings as gifts.

Tangerines are the easiest citrus fruit to peel, and for that reason, they're nicknamed "the easy peelers."

The tangelo is a cross between a tangerine and a grapefruit.

springtime citrus cakelette creations

ingredients

2 eggs
6 T unsalted butter, melted
½ C sugar
½ C milk
2 T olive oil
1 ½ C all-purpose flour (or gluten-free flour)
3 T cornstarch
¾ tsp baking soda
¼ tsp baking powder
¼ tsp salt

choose any kinds of winter citrus (try at least 3!):
grapefruit
lemon
lime
orange (any kind)
tangelo
tangerine

preheat+crack+whisk

Preheat oven to 350 degrees F. Crack **2 eggs** and add to a mixing bowl. Whisk the eggs with **6 tablespoons of melted butter (room-temp, not hot), ½ cup of sugar, ½ cup of milk,** and **2 tablespoons of olive oil.**

measure+sift+zest+juice

Measure and add **1½ cups of flour** and **3 tablespoons of cornstarch** to a second mixing bowl. Add ¼ **teaspoon of baking powder,** ¾ **teaspoon of baking soda,** and ¼ **teaspoon of salt.** Use a whisk to mix and sift out any lumps! Then wash and zest the outer, colored peel of **3 citrus fruits.** Set the zest aside. Cut each citrus fruit in half and squeeze the juice into a separate bowl.

combine+stir+bake

Combine wet ingredients and dry ingredients. Stir gently until all traces of flour disappear. Kids can add in citrus zest to the whole batch, or separate the batter and make different flavors. Have them also add about **2 tablespoons of squeezed citrus juice** to the batter and mix, too. Save leftover citrus juice for the Sweet-Tart Citrus Glaze. Divide the batter into a greased muffin pan and bake until an inserted toothpick comes out clean and cakelettes have turned golden brown, about 20 to 25 minutes. Drizzle with *Sweet-Tart Citrus Glaze* and *Citrus Peel Confetti!*

sweet-tart citrus glaze
+ citrus peel confetti

ingredients

1 C full-fat Greek yogurt

4 T citrus juice

powdered sugar to taste

measure + add + whisk

Measure and add **1 cup of yogurt** into a bowl (or divide it into 2 to 3 bowls and make different flavors of glazes!). Add a total of **4 tablespoons of citrus juice** to your cup of yogurt, divided by however many flavors you're making. Add **sugar to taste** to make sweeter, starting with a teaspoon. Whisk! Drizzle glaze over baked and cooled cakelettes and sprinkle with extra reserved citrus zest (this is your *Citrus Peel Confetti!*). YUM!

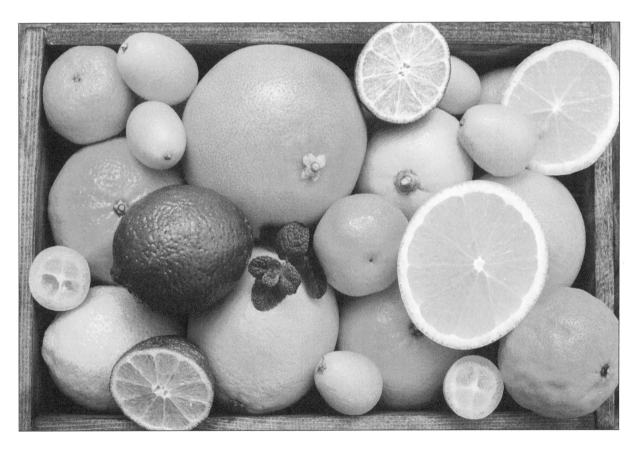

easy breezy citrus-ade

ingredients

2 oranges

1 grapefruit

4 lemons

5 limes

¼ to ½ C sugar

ice

squeeze+add

Use your muscles to squeeze every bit of **juice from 2 oranges, 1 grapefruit, 4 lemons,** and **5 limes.** Add the juice, **¼ to ½ cups of sugar** and 3 cups of cold water to your blender.

blend+strain+pour

Blend on high for 15 seconds. Taste and add more sugar if needed. Pour into small cups over **ice** and CHEERS!

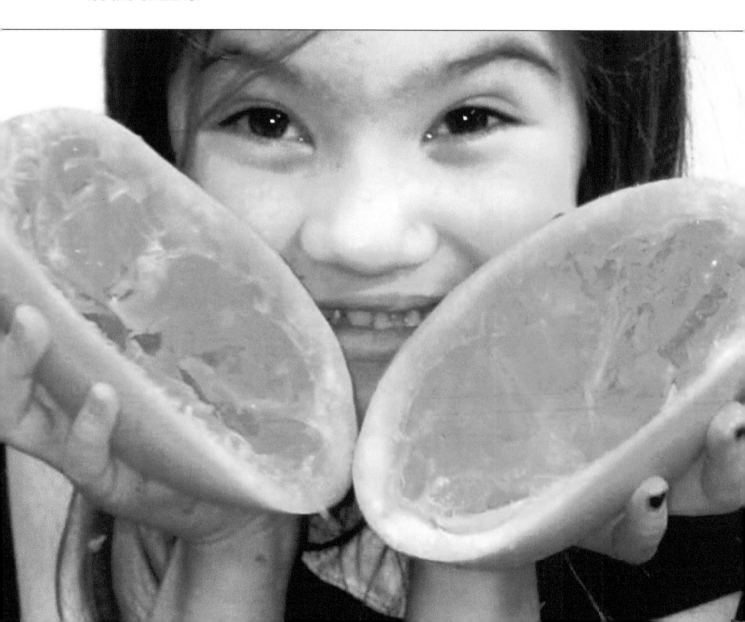

cultivating 'COOL'inary curiosity in kids™

thyme for a fun activity

Farmers Market
Family Scavenger Hunt

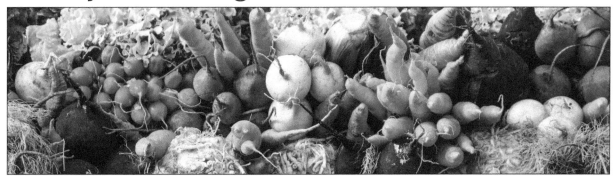

The next time you and your family are at a farmers market (or even at the grocery store), play this fun scavenger hunt to explore all the wonderful and delicious items available!

- Find a **green** vegetable **you have never tried before**

- Find a **fruit and/or vegetable** for each **color of the rainbow**

- Learn the **name of a new flower** or herb

- Find something that **grows on a vine**

- Find something that **grows under the ground**

- Find something that **grows on trees**

- **Ask a vendor** their favorite produce they grow

- Buy a **new flavor of jam, jelly, or preserves** you've never tried before

- Find **seeds** that can be planted in a garden

- Buy **5 farm-fresh ingredients** you could use to make a **salad**

- Buy **5 farm-fresh ingredients** you could use on a **pizza**

- Find the **biggest vegetable at the market**

- Find an **ingredient** that would surprise or **"freak out" your family!**

- Find **flowers** you could use as a **surprise gift** for someone special

FUN CHALLENGE: Try to find a fruit and/or vegetable for every letter of the alphabet!

SUMMERTIME

Ahh, summertime! Eggplant, tomatoes, cucumbers, bell peppers, strawberries, blueberries, and lettuce all practically transform themselves straight from the garden into these beautiful, mouthwatering, and summery recipes with minimal effort from you and your kids. And when the weather's warm, we all belong outside spending time with our families!

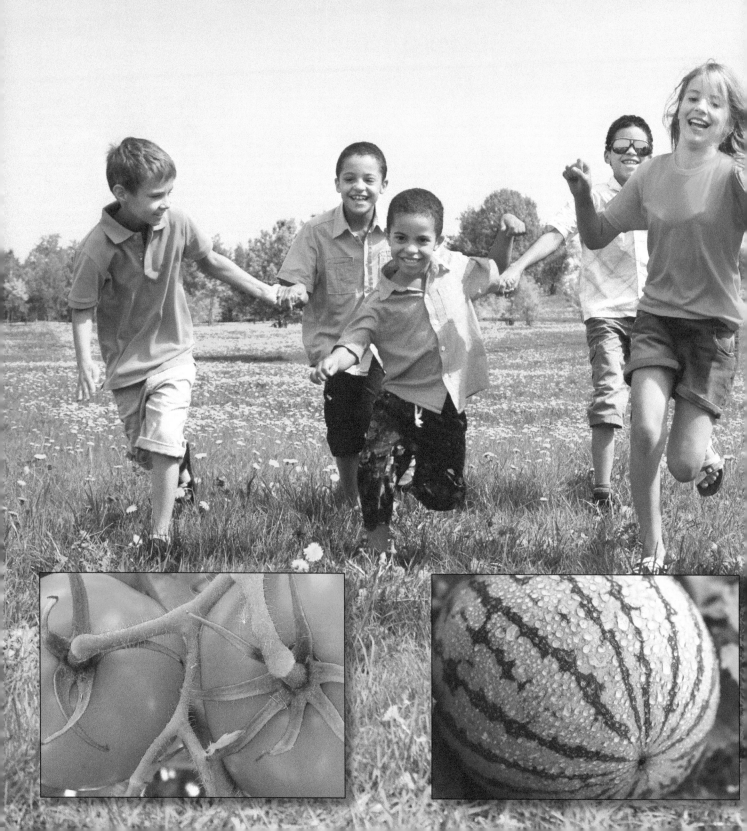

"Live in the sunshine, swim the sea, drink the wild air." *- Ralph Waldo Emerson*

A life without love is like a year without summer. *- Swedish Proverb*

Laugh Time: What do monsters like to eat in the summer? I Scream!

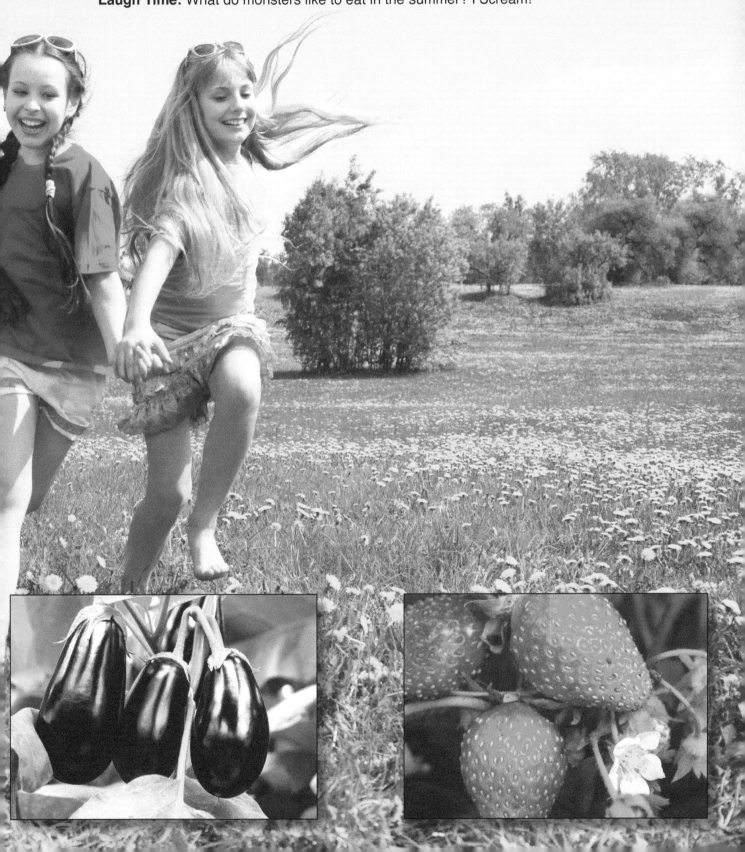

Scrumptious Summertime Blueberry Lemon Ricotta Pancakes
+ Kid-Made Blueberry Butter

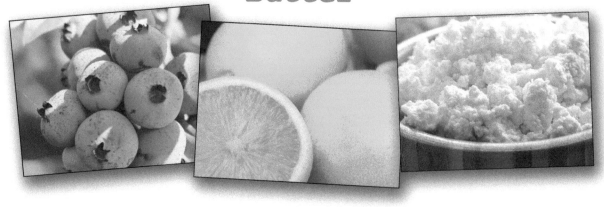

fun food story:

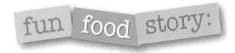

Pancake History

Pancakes are a universal food found in many variations from Africa to Asia to Europe and South America. A pancake is a thin, flat cake made from batter and cooked on a hot, flat surface such as a griddle or fry pan. Most pancakes are quick breads, meaning the rise comes from baking powder or soda, not yeast. However, some pancake variations do rely on yeast or fermented butter. Depending on the region, pancakes may be served with a variety of fillings or toppings including fruit, syrup, jam, or even different kinds of meat, and they can be eaten at any time of day.

Archaeological evidence suggests that pancakes are most likely one of the earliest and most widespread types of cereal food eaten. It is believed seed flours were mixed with protein-based liquids and cooked on hot stones or shallow pots over a fire.

The pancake's shape and structure vary worldwide. In Germany, Hungary, and Israel, pancakes can be made from potatoes. A crêpe is a French variety of thin pancake cooked on one or both sides in a special crêpe pan to achieve a network of fine bubbles often compared to lace.

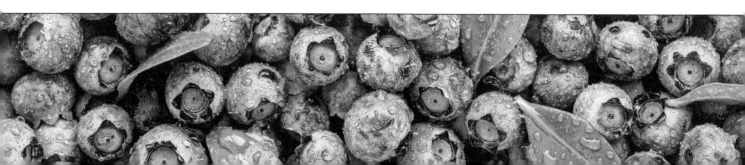

The featured ingredient: Blueberries!

★ **Native Americans once called them "star berries"** because the five points of a blueberry blossom makes a star shape.

★ **Blueberry juice had medicinal value for Native Americans** and was used to treat persistent coughs and other illnesses.

★ **The traditional blue paint used in the homes of Shakers was made from blueberry skins,** sage blossoms, indigo, and milk.

★ **America's favorite muffin is,** of course, blueberry.

★ **Blueberries are one of the only natural foods** that are truly blue in color.

★ **The pale, powder-like, protective coating** on the skin of blueberries is called "bloom."

★ **Blueberries contain more antioxidants** than most other fruits or vegetables!

★ **A blueberry extract diet improves** balance, coordination, short-term memory, and eyesight.

★ **The blueberry industry of North America** ships over 500 metric tons of fresh berries to Japan each year and over 100 metric tons to Iceland.

★ **Maine is the blueberry production capital of North America** and produces almost 100 percent of all berries harvested in the country.

● ●

summertime blueberry lemon ricotta pancakes

ingredients

1½ C all-purpose flour
3 T baking powder
1 tsp ground nutmeg
½ tsp salt
4 T sugar
2 lemons (reserve juice and zest)

½ C fresh ricotta cheese
1½ C fresh or frozen (thawed) blueberries
4 eggs
1⅓ C milk
oil or unsalted butter (for cooking)

dry measure

Measure and combine **1½ cups of flour, 3 tablespoons of baking powder, 1 teaspoon of nutmeg, ½ teaspoon of salt, and 4 tablespoon sugar** in a small bowl.

wash+zest+squeeze

Wash **2 lemons,** and using a fine cheese grater, zest the peel of the lemons (only the yellow part) and squeeze the juice. Reserve the lemon juice and zest.

wet measure

In a large bowl, measure and whisk together ½ **cup of ricotta cheese, 1½ cups of blueberries, 4 eggs, 1⅓ cups of milk,** and **reserved lemon juice and lemon zest**.

fold+cook

Lightly whisk or fold the flour mixture into the wet ingredients until just combined. Brush a hot griddle with oil or butter. For each pancake, pour approximately 1 to 2 tablespoons batter onto the griddle and cook on both sides until light golden brown. Repeat until no batter remains. Makes about 24 to 28 silver-dollar-sized pancakes.

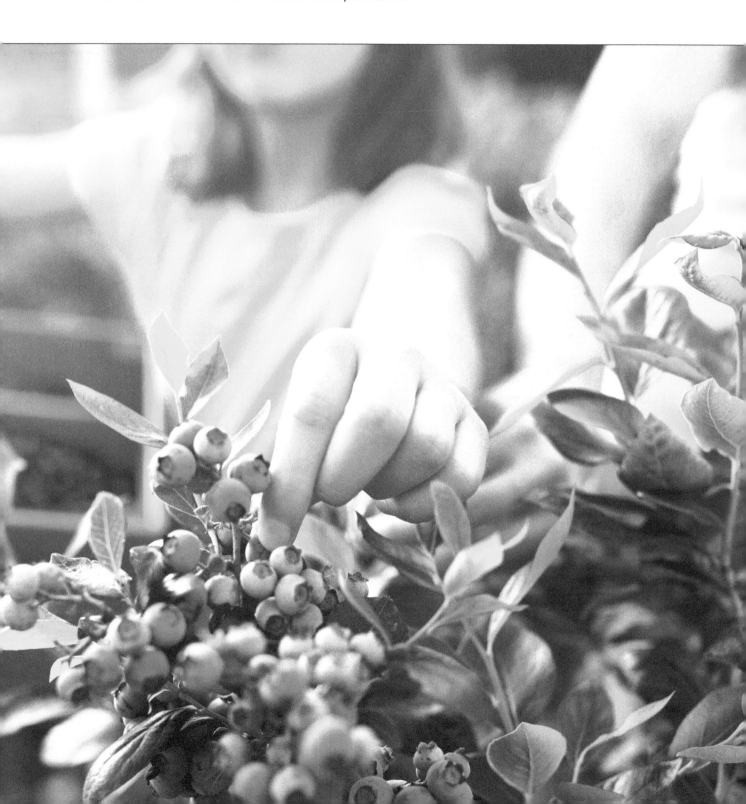

kid-made blueberry butter

ingredients

1 pint heavy whipping cream

1 orange (zested)

1 T blueberry jam

pinch salt

zest!+add!+shake!

Find a glass jar with a tight-fitting lid. Fill jar ½ **full of heavy whipping cream.** Wash and zest **1 orange** (orange part only) with a fine cheese grater and add ½ **teaspoon of orange zest** to the whipping cream with **a pinch of salt.** Screw on lid tightly. Shake, shake, shake, shake until the cream becomes butter. This step may take 5 minutes or so. Drain off excess liquid from butter. Add **1 tablespoon of blueberry jam** and mix into the fresh butter AFTER it has been made. Add extra honey to taste and serve on top of the *Scrumptious Summertime Blueberry Lemon Ricotta Pancakes.* YUM! YUM!

Let's Finish with a Laugh!

What do you get when you cross ice, chocolate, a big blueberry, a giant banana, and cold milk?
The world's best Sundae!

Why did the blueberry stop in the middle of the road?
Because it ran out of juice...

What did the blueberry say to the other blueberry?
You're a blueberry.

What is a ghost's favorite fruit?
A Boo-Berry!

Tantalizing Thai Lettuce Wraps + Sweet and Sour Mushrooms
+ Thai Lime Shakes

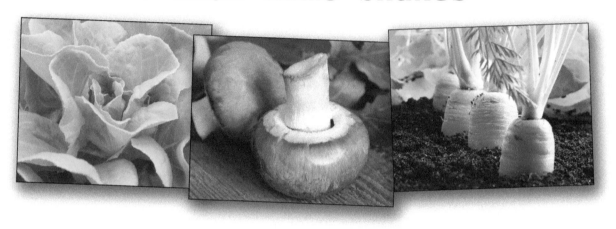

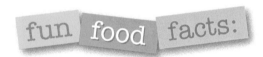

The History of Lettuce Wraps

Delicious lettuce wraps are a typical Southeast Asian specialty. According to customs, lettuce wraps were eaten by women of the Thai Royal Court who had been taken as maids or ladies of the court. On the first full moon of the lunar year, lettuce wraps are eaten for good luck. Lettuce wraps are also gaining popularity outside of Asia and are being served at restaurants all over the world.

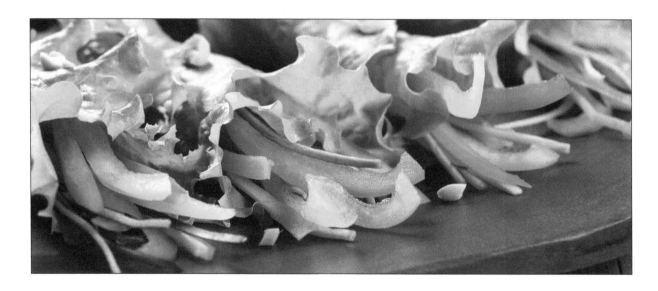

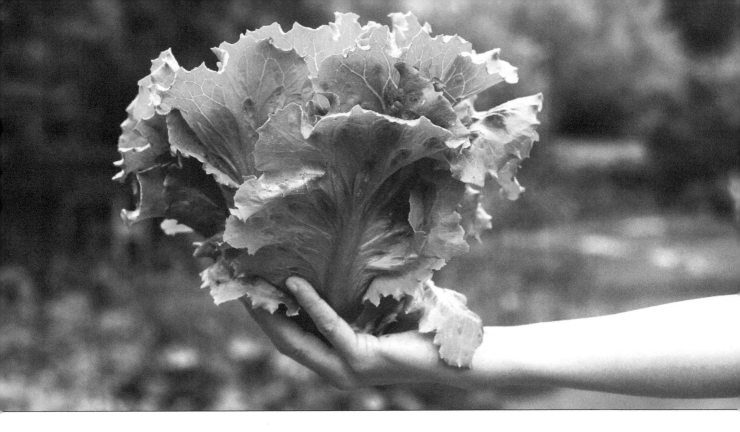

The featured ingredient: Lettuce!

★ **Where modern lettuce comes from is not exactly known,** but it is thought to have originated from a wild lettuce in the temperate, mountainous areas around southwestern Asia and the Middle East. Also, people in ancient Egypt cultivated lettuce around 6,000 years ago. Paintings in royal tombs show us that consuming lettuce was a part of the ancient Egyptian diet.

★ **Lettuce is one of the most popular salad vegetables**. There are many different varieties, shapes, sizes, and colors of lettuce.

★ **The name "iceberg" lettuce comes from the preservation method that was used at the beginning of the 20th century in California.** When refrigerators were not available, large quantities of ice were used to prevent spoilage of lettuce while it traveled via train to markets. Carriages were filled with icebergs that floated on top of the lettuce. Iceberg lettuce is the most popular and most cultivated variety of lettuce in the US. Unfortunately, it is the LEAST nutritious lettuce.

★ **Both the English name (lettuce) and the Latin name (lactuca sativa)** are derived from "lac," the Latin word for "milk," referring to the plant's milky juice.

★ **The DARKER the lettuce leaf, the MORE nutritious it is.** Any varieties of lettuce with dark green leaves are a good source of beta-carotene.

★ **Lettuce is about 95% water,** so it is hydrating and refreshing!

★ **Lettuce provides dietary fiber, vitamins A, B9, C, and folate and minerals such as calcium, iron, and copper.** Fibers are concentrated in the ribs, whereas minerals and vitamins are found in the leafy part of the lettuce.

tantalizing thai lettuce wraps with sweet+sour mushrooms

ingredients

for sweet+sour mushrooms:
8 oz mushrooms
1½ T oil
1 T soy sauce
1 large head butter lettuce

for dipping sauce:
1 small garlic clove
½ C rice vinegar
¼ C sugar
1 tsp salt

slice+sauté

Make the mushroom filling! While the dipping sauce is cooling, have your kids chop and slice **8 oz of mushrooms** into little bits. Heat **1½ tablespoons of oil** in a skillet over high heat. Add the mushrooms and toss them for several minutes in the skillet until they absorb the oil and start to brown. Add **1 tablespoon of soy sauce** and continue sautéing the mushrooms until most (or all) of the soy sauce has been absorbed and the mushrooms are cooked through. Remove from heat and transfer mushrooms to a bowl.

mince+measure+cook+toss

Time to make the dipping sauce! Have your kids start by mincing **1 garlic clove** and add to a medium saucepan on the stovetop. Then have them measure and combine ½ **cup of rice vinegar**, ¼ **cup of sugar, 1 teaspoon of salt** into the saucepan. Cook on medium heat, stirring with a wooden spoon, until the sugar and salt melt (the sauce will become clear). Remove the sauce from the heat and allow to cool slightly. Add 2 tablespoons of the dipping sauce to the mushrooms and toss.

chop+slice+grate+tear+pre-cook

Now have your kids chop, slice, tear, and grate whichever fresh and tasty lettuce wrap fillings they want to try from the following list (choose at least four!) and set each in a separate bowl. If also using rice noodles as a filling, pre-cook on the stovetop according to package directions.

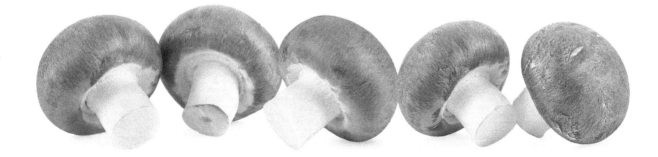

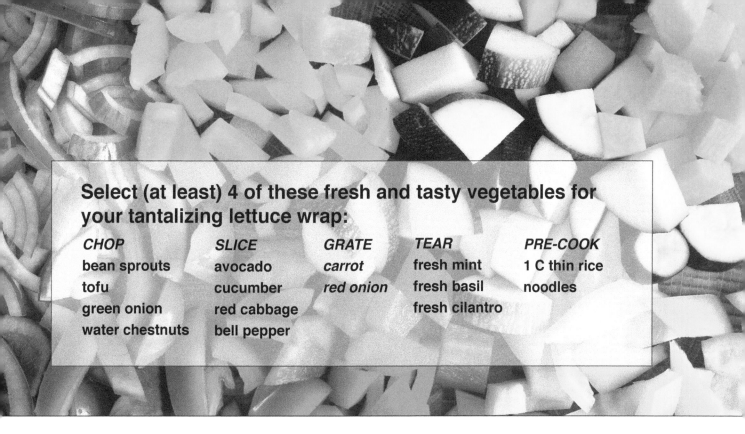

Select (at least) 4 of these fresh and tasty vegetables for your tantalizing lettuce wrap:

CHOP	*SLICE*	*GRATE*	*TEAR*	*PRE-COOK*
bean sprouts	avocado	*carrot*	fresh mint	1 C thin rice
tofu	cucumber	*red onion*	fresh basil	noodles
green onion	red cabbage		fresh cilantro	
water chestnuts	bell pepper			

separate+wash

Separate the leaves on **1 head of butter lettuce.** Wash under cold water and set aside to dry.

fill+wrap

Kids can make their own lettuce wraps when the mushrooms are ready to eat! To serve, have kids take 1 butter lettuce leaf at a time and spoon a tablespoon of the slightly cooled mushroom mixture into the center of the leaf. Add the prepped vegetables and fold, wrapping the lettuce around the filling. Serve with the extra dipping sauce. *Say aroi dee*, "delicious" in Thai!

● ●

thai lime shakes

ingredients

2 to 3 limes

1 C crushed ice

pinch salt

3 T sugar/agave/honey/stevia (to taste)

combine+blend

Have your kids juice **2 to 3 limes** right into the blender and then have them add **1 cup of crushed ice**, ½ cup of water, and **3 tablespoons of sugar/agave/honey (or stevia to taste)**. Add a **pinch of salt** if you like! Blend until slushy. Sample to see if it needs more sugar to cut the sour taste from the lime juice. Serve and ENJOY!

Radical Ratatouille
+ Fabulous Fresh French Bread Knots + Blender Basil Lemon Sorbet

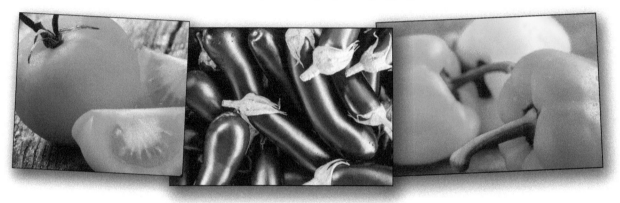

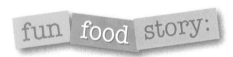

fun food story:

I had a transformational bite of food at Alain Ducasse's famous restaurant, *La Bastide de Moustiers*, in the south of France with my soon-to-be-husband in 1997. It was one of those moments that I will never forget, and I know that it helped shaped my love of food and cooking which eventually led me to Sticky Fingers Cooking.

That bite of food was ratatouille, while on the restaurant's balcony on a late July afternoon. I continue to sit on that balcony many times each year. In my mind. I am also very dear, very close, personal friends with the famed California Chef Alice Waters. In my mind.

Ratatouille (Rat-at-TOO-ee): The word comes from the French term *touiller*, which means to toss food. This ratatouille recipe is inspired by Alice Waters' farm-to-table, one-skillet dish, tossing food together, and my lovely memory of the south of France in the summer of 1997.

Most of us have seen the movie *Ratatouille*. This movie was released in 2007, 10 years after my first bite of Alain Ducasse's ratatouille. The movie's central theme is about a rat named Remy, whose great desire is to be a Parisian gourmet chef. We begin with Remy's journey, which starts entirely by accident and leads to adventure. At the tail end of the movie, Anton Ego, the feared, cold-hearted food critic, is disarmed and positively undone when he takes a bite of Remy's ratatouille and is transported back to his mother's kitchen, a place where he felt happy and loved as a child. I may not be a feared and cold-hearted food critic, but I did experience that transformational feeling while sitting on that balcony in France in 1997 eating ratatouille, just like Ego did.

Maybe your children will feel a spark when they create a new recipe at home with you, and maybe there will be an "a-ha moment" when they realize that they actually *do* like to eat eggplant. Maybe they will learn to love the pleasure and the magical memory that the art of good cooking and eating provides us. Maybe! *Merci beaucoup*, Alain, Alice, and Remy the Rat.

Have fun + happy, healthy cooking! - Chef Erin

● ●

The featured ingredient: Eggplant!

When you see an eggplant for the first time, what comes to mind? Stop! Don't touch it! The deadly "mad apple" will be the end of you! "Danger" is what most of the modern world thought for centuries when they encountered this odd-looking plant. They had good reason to think this, though, since eggplant belongs to the nightshade family whose members include poisonous plants like Datura (aka Jimsonweed) and Belladonna (aka Deadly Nightshade).

★ **The eggplant is considered a vegetable but is really a fruit,** (technically, it's a BERRY!!).

★ **Early varieties of eggplant were round and white, they resembled chicken eggs.** That's how they got their name... EGGPLANT!

★ **Eggplants are related to potatoes, tomatoes, peppers, and (even) tobacco.**

★ **Thomas Jefferson brought the eggplant to the United States, where the eggplant was only used as a table ornament (like flowers)** until the 20th century. People thought they were poisonous!

★ **Eggplant is good for you!** It helps to keep your immune system strong and is also a source of vitamin B, folic acid, fiber, and potassium

★ **When buying eggplant, look for one that is heavy and has a smooth, shiny, deep-purple skin.** Squeeze the eggplant gently with a finger and then let go: The eggplant will bounce back smoothly if it is fresh. The eggplant should feel heavy.

The eggplant itself, during its immature growth stage, contains toxins that can cause illness. Fear not! Nightshade plants also include yummy potatoes and tomatoes!

Eggplants are from India but became very popular in China. We do know that the Emperors of China enjoyed them as early as 600 BCE. Fashionable ladies of 600 BCE in China used a dye made from eggplant skins to stain their teeth black, which was considered stylish (I can't think why—it would look pretty yucky to me)! At this time, the rest of the world had NEVER seen an eggplant.

Eggplants then made their way around the world as a "toxic" ornamental decoration on the tables of Spanish, Greek, and Portuguese explorer ships for centuries. People were afraid of them!

In the 1600s, King Louis XIV of France, who took great interest in impressing his royal dining companions with new plant foods, became the first person in France to introduce

eggplant into his garden. Eggplant did not impress the King's guests at first. At that time, eggplants were described as: "fruits as large as pears, but with bad qualities." The urban legend of the time was that eating eggplant caused fever and epilepsy. You have to realize that at the time, the eggplants we are talking about were not the beautiful purple shapes they are now. They were often small, yellow-brown, egg-shaped fruits. He cooked them and served them to his royal dinner guests, and guess what?! They didn't get sick! It was amazing! After some research, he realized that once they mature, eggplants are pretty delicious!

After King Louis started serving it at royal dinners, eggplant became the hot item of the time. All the countries were talking about this mysterious fruit that could only be eaten at certain times of its life or else it would cause illness.

It became so popular that Thomas Jefferson, the 3rd president of the United States and an avid botanist, decided to bring it over to the USA with many other of the world's exotic plants to make his garden more impressive.

radical ratatouille

ingredients

1 medium eggplant	3 ripe tomatoes
1 tsp salt + pinch	5 to 6 T olive oil
2 to 4 stalks green onions	big pinch mild chili powder
4 garlic cloves	1 big pinch sugar
2 red/yellow bell peppers	6 fresh basil leaves
2 medium zucchinis	½ to ¾ C grated Parmesan cheese

cut+drain

Cut **1 eggplant** into cubes and toss with **1 teaspoon + pinch of salt** . Set the cubes in a colander to drain for about 5 to 10 minutes. This helps remove the bitter taste from the eggplant.

chop+slice

Chop and slice up **2 to 4 green onion stalks, 4 garlic cloves, 2 bell peppers, 2 zucchinis,** and **3 tomatoes** into very small bits.

heat+pat

Heat **2 tablespoons of olive oil** in a skillet over medium heat on your stovetop. Pat the salted eggplant dry with paper towels and add to the skillet. Cook over medium heat, stirring frequently, until golden. Add a bit more oil if the eggplant begins to stick to the bottom of the pan. Remove the eggplant when done and set aside.

drizzle+pinch

In the same skillet, drizzle 2 tablespoons of olive oil. Add the chopped green onions and cook for about 3 to 5 minutes, or until soft. Add the chopped garlic, **1 pinch of chili powder, 1 pinch of sugar,** and a pinch of salt. Cook for 2 to 3 minutes and then stir in the chopped peppers. Cook for a few minutes more and then stir in the chopped zucchini. Cook for a few more minutes and then stir in the chopped tomatoes. Finally, cook for 2 minutes longer and then stir in the pre-cooked eggplant. Continue to cook until all of the vegetables are tender.

season+stir+top

Taste and adjust the seasoning with salt, if needed. Stir in **6 fresh chopped basil leaves** and a drizzle more of olive oil. Top with ½ **to ¾ cups Parmesan cheese,** to taste. Serve warm or cool with the bread.

● ●

fabulous fresh french bread knots

ingredients

butter or oil (for greasing)
1 C + 2 T warm water
⅓ C olive oil
2 T active dry yeast
¼ C sugar

1 egg
½ to ¾ C grated Parmesan cheese
3 C all-purpose flour
1 tsp salt

preheat+grease

Preheat your oven to 375 degrees F and grease a muffin pan with butter or oil.

pour+rest

In a bowl, pour **1 cup + 2 tablespoons of warm water, ⅓ cup of olive oil, 2 tablespoons of yeast, and ¼ cup of sugar.** Allow the mixture to rest for 8 to 15 minutes.

whip+stir

Crack **1 egg** into the bowl and whip the egg with the yeast mixture. Stir in ½ **to ¾ cup of Parmesan cheese.**

measure+mix

In a new bowl, measure and **mix 3 cups of flour** and **1 teaspoon of salt** together. Then, ½ cup at a time, add flour/salt mixture into your yeast mixture, mixing well until a dough is formed.

shape+bake

Shape the dough into about 12 balls and let the dough rest and rise for at least 20 minutes and up to 1 hour — the longer the better! After your dough has rested, place the balls in the wells of your greased muffin pan. Bake for 30 to 40 minutes in your preheated oven, or until the tops are just golden brown.

● ●

blender basil lemon sorbet

ingredients

1 C water (boiling)

4 to 6 fresh basil leaves

¼ C sugar

2 to 4 lemons (for juicing)

2 to 4 C ice

tear+steep

Start by making a basil simple syrup 'tea'. Boil **1 cup of water** and tear up **4 to 6 fresh basil leaves.** Add **1/4 cup of sugar** along with the torn basil leaves into a bowl or heat-proof cup. Carefully add the hot water to sugar, stir, and let sit until sugar has dissolved.

squeeze+blend

Squeeze in the juice from **2 to 4 lemons** into your blender and then add your basil simple syrup 'tea' and **2 to 4 cups of ice.** Blend until thick (adding more ice, if needed) and serve with spoons!

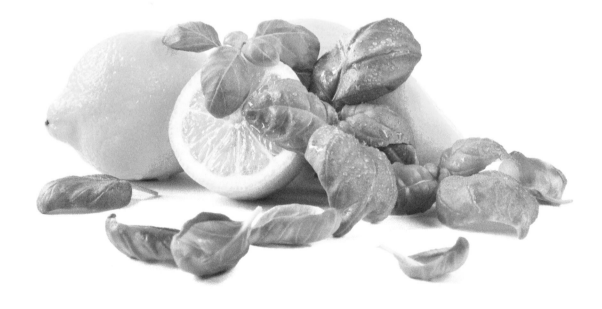

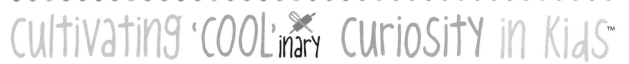

cultivating 'COOL'inary curiosity in Kids™

Lovely Leftovers Stamp Art

ingredients:

leftover raw veggies such as:
broccoli
cauliflower
parsnip
potato
bottom of celery
bottom of romaine heart
bottom of bell pepper

supplies:

small knife and/or cookie cutters
cutting board
washable paint or ink pad
paper

directions:

🚜 **Go on a refrigerator raid to select which leftover fruits and vegetables you'd like to use for stamping.** Try to choose leftovers that have an interesting shape. If you're using leftover veggies such as parsnips or potatoes, you can cut them into fun shapes like stars or hearts.

🚜 **Cut the leftovers into handheld sizes, with the "stamp" side being as flat as possible.** You can also try to use cookie cutters to cut out your shape on softer foods like zucchini or squash!

🚜 **Stamp your shaped leftovers into your ink pad or onto a plate of washable paint** (you may need to rotate your stamp in the ink or paint a bit for fuller coverage) and press down firmly onto your paper.

🚜 **Lift up and see what beautiful shapes you've made!** Who knew leftovers could be so versatile?

Let's Finish with a Laugh!

What kind of vegetable likes to look at animals?
A zoo-chini!

How do you fix a broken tomato?
Tomato paste!

Crisp Mezzelune
Strawberry Ravioli
Whipped Sweet Ricotta + Fresh
Strawberry Sgroppino
Milkshakes

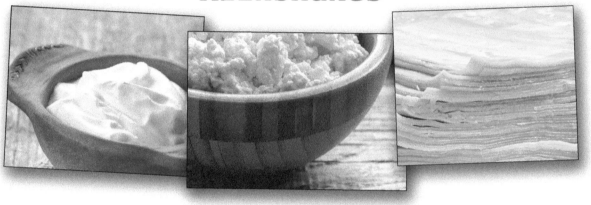

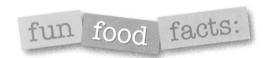

The History of Ravioli

Derived from an Italian word meaning "to wrap," ravioli practically hold their own universe, with such a tremendous variation in the fillings. Most say that true ravioli should not contain any meat, a valid claim. This dish dates back to 14th century Italy, where meat was often expensive and inaccessible to most, so people stuffed ravioli with wild greens and sometimes simple cheeses, if they had it.

Stuffed pasta has a long history and, depending on the region of Italy, a number of recipe varieties. You could travel all over the country and never eat the same stuffed pasta twice because each region has its own form and stuffings.

A century ago in Italy, meat- and vegetable-filled pastas often were an indication of one's economic status. The affluent could afford to eat meat-filled pastas year round while the less affluent generally ate vegetable-filled pastas throughout the year; though both opted for meatless varieties on Fridays during the Christian season of Lent.

The featured ingredient: Strawberries!

★ **Strawberries are the only fruit to have seeds on the outside of the skin!** The average strawberry holds about 200 seeds.

★ **Strawberries are actually members of the rose (Rosaceae) family,** along with apples, pears, and even almonds!

★ **The largest strawberries in history weighed over 8 oz** and were the size of a big apple!

★ **Although strawberries have grown in the wild for thousands of years,** Europeans started cultivating the plant during the Renaissance period.

★ **It is believed that strawberries derive their name from the words "strewn berries,"** referring to how easily the plant spreads and produces runners.

★ **Strawberries are high in vitamin C, fiber, folate, and potassium** yet relatively low in calories. They also are rich in antioxidants, making them a heart-healthy fruit.

★ **According to folklore, strawberries were great at matchmaking!** It was believed that if you split a double strawberry and shared it with someone you liked, you would fall in love with each other. In France, strawberries were thought to be a love potion; soup made of strawberries, thinned sour cream, and powdered sugar was served to newlyweds.

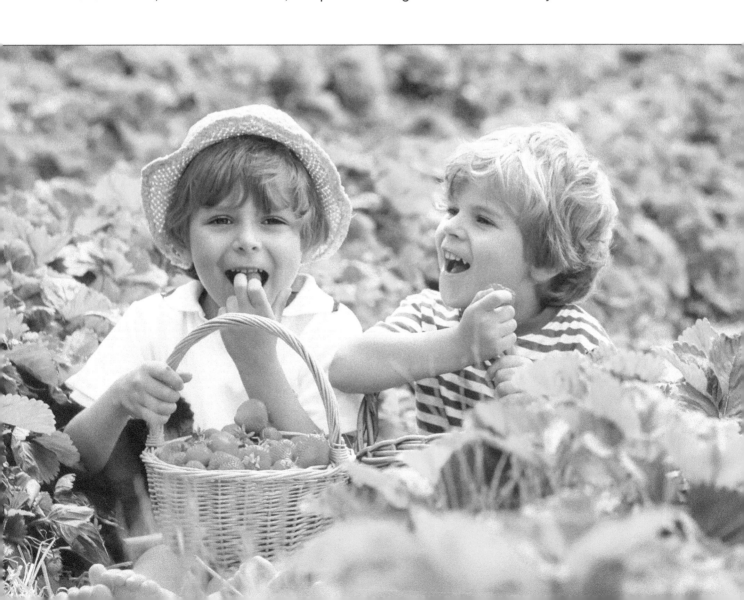

crisp mezzelune strawberry ravioli

ingredients

1 lemon (for zesting and juicing)	2 tsp cornstarch
½ pint fresh strawberries (about 6 to 8 large strawberries)	2 T ricotta cheese
pinch salt	24 wonton wrappers (sub Asian rice paper for GF)
¼ C sugar	olive oil (for cooking)

zest+chop

Zest the **rind of 1 lemon** and set to the side for *Whipped Sweet Ricotta* recipe. Chop ½ **pint of fresh strawberries** (about 6 to 8 large strawberries) into small bits — the smaller, the better!

pinch+measure+squeeze

Add the strawberries to a bowl with **a pinch of salt, ¼ cup of sugar, 2 teaspoons of cornstarch, 2 tablespoons of ricotta cheese,** and ½ **tablespoon of fresh lemon juice** (from your zested lemon!).

mix+macerate

Mix the filling together until the berries are coated. Next 'macerate' the strawberry mixture (a method of preparation where an ingredient softens or breaks down by being soaking in a liquid) and let the mixture sit for at least two minutes or up to three hours.

cut+trace+fill+seal

Using either the lid of a jar or a round cookie cutter, make circles out of your **wonton wrappers.** Have kids dip a clean finger in a bowl of water and trace the water around the edges of the circular wonton wrapper. Place about **1 teaspoon of strawberry filing** in the center of the wonton and fold over one side to make a half-moon (mezzelune) shaped pocket. Press the edges down to seal, making sure to push out all of the air in the center, as the strawberry filling will seep out if there is too much air in the ravioli when you cook them.

fry+crisp

Heat a non-stick skillet on your stovetop over medium heat and add a big lug of **olive oil**. Slip the ravioli into the skillet, without any water, cover and cook until browned on one side, about 2 minutes. Flip and cook on the second side until browned and crisp. Fry up as many ravioli as you can, setting them all to the side on a plate to cool. Serve with *Whipped Sweet Ricotta* and sprinkle a little extra sugar on top, if desired!

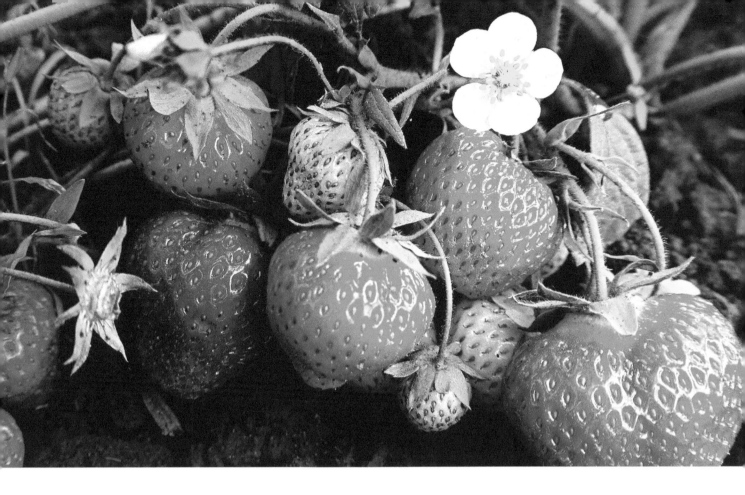

whipped sweet ricotta

ingredients

½ C ricotta cheese

3 T sugar

1 tsp lemon zest

1 tsp lemon juice

measure+whisk+whip

Measure ½ **cup of ricotta cheese, 3 tablespoons of sugar, 1 teaspoon of lemon zest,** and **1 teaspoon of lemon juice** into a bowl. Whisk and whip together. Serve a dollop of whipped ricotta with the crisp strawberry ravioli — dip, eat, and enjoy!

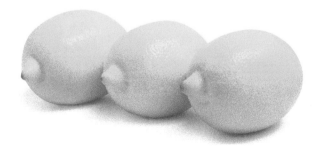

fresh strawberry sgroppino milkshakes

ingredients

½ pint fresh strawberries (about 6-8 large strawberries)

1 T lemon juice

1 T honey or sugar

2 T ricotta cheese

1½ C sparkling water

1½ C lemon sorbet

chop+squeeze+blend

Chop ½ **pint of fresh strawberries** (about 6-8 large strawberries) and add to your blender or a pitcher for use with a hand blender. Squeeze **1 tablespoon of lemon juice** into the blender/pitcher. Add **1 tablespoon of honey or sugar** and **2 tablespoons of ricotta cheese.** Blend everything together until the berries are a smooth puree.

measure+whisk

Measure and add **1½ cups of sparkling water** and **1½ cups of lemon sorbet** to berry puree in a pitcher. Quickly whisk the ingredients together by hand until a light and frothy mousse forms. Be careful not to over-mix or it will separate and become limp and soupy. Spoon the mixture into cups and serve immediately!

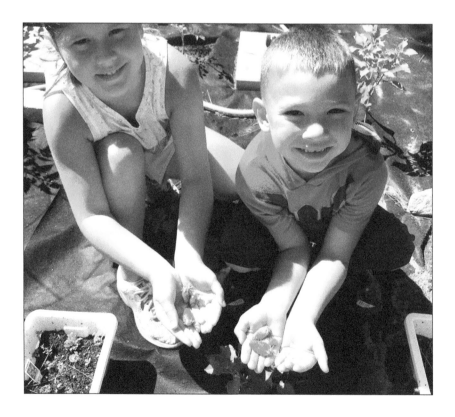

Let's Finish with a Laugh!

Why was the farmer in jail?
For armed stROBBERY!

What is a scarecrow's favorite fruit?
Straw-berries!

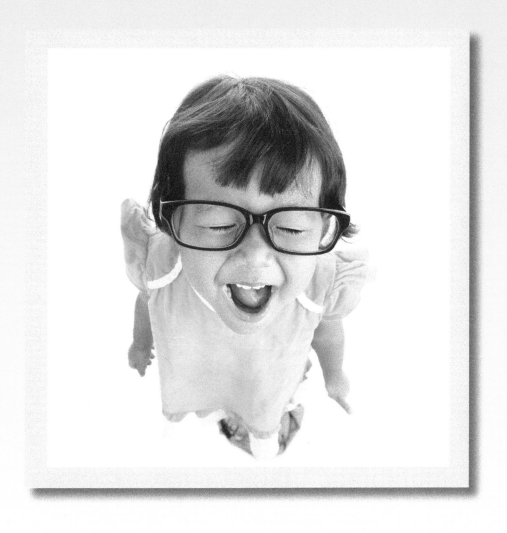

Glorious Garden Gazpacho with Corn Relish +
Cheesy Herby Flatbread
+ Easy Grape
Granizados

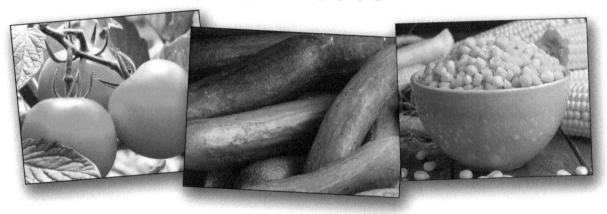

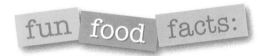

Gazpacho!

Gazpacho is a delicious, cold, tomato-based, raw vegetable soup!
This yummy soup originated in southern Spain. Gazpacho remained popular with farmers as a way to cool off during the summer and as a simple way to make a cool, easily eaten lunch with locally available ingredients such as fresh vegetables, olive oil, and bread.

The featured ingredient: Tomatoes!

★ **Tomatoes were originally cultivated by the Aztec and Incan peoples in the Americas as early as 700 CE.** Explorers brought the tomato seed to back to Europe in the 1500s, though northern countries were not as fond of the tomato.

★ **The British actually believed the fruit was poisonous, and that fear spread to the American colonies.** It wasn't until the 1800s that people began accepting and regularly cultivating tomatoes.

★ **The tomatoes are related to the potatoes, peppers, eggplants, and petunias.**

★ **There are thousands of different tomato varieties,** including beefsteak, heirloom, roma, and cherry.

★ **Tomatoes are a very good source of the antioxidant lycopene** as well as vitamins A, C, K, and potassium.

★ **Green tomatoes are harvested before being ripe!** Consumed fresh, they have a rather unpleasant, sour taste. However, when cooked, as in fried green tomatoes, they have a sharp, sweeter flavor.

● ●

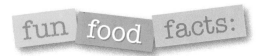

The featured ingredient: Garlic!

★ **Garlic is a relative of the onion** and adds depth and flavor to many dishes.

★ **Garlic has been used for medicinal purposes for thousands of years by ancient civilizations** like the Greeks, Egyptians, Babylonians, and Chinese. Scientists today now know the sulfur compounds present in garlic are responsible for most of its health benefits.

★ **Garlic is among the oldest cultivated plants in the world.**

★ **The ancient Egyptians worshipped garlic,** and it was once so valuable it was used as money.

★ **To rid your hands of garlic smell, wash them thoroughly with cold water and then rub them on a chrome faucet.**

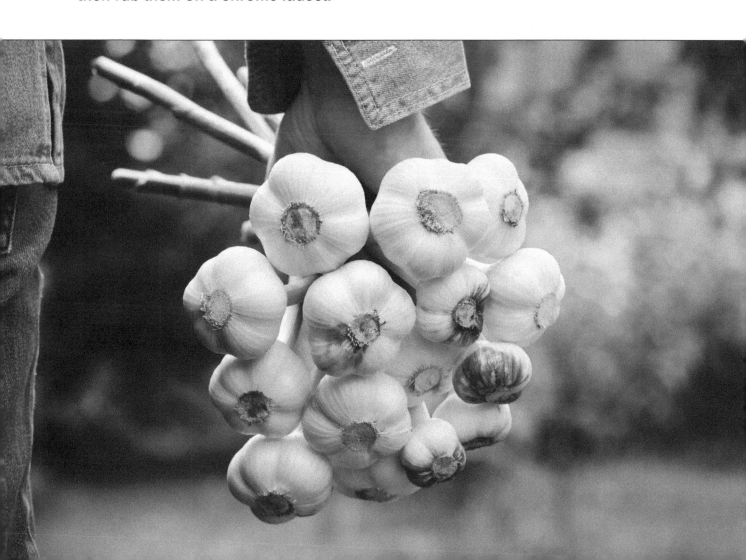

glorious garden gazpacho

ingredients

¼ baguette
½ C extra virgin cold-pressed olive oil (+ more for drizzling)
1 to 2 T white wine vinegar
8 ripe tomatoes
2 tsp sugar

1 garlic clove
3 tsp + sea salt + more to taste
2 small English cucumbers
2 T fresh tarragon
1 C fresh or frozen sweet corn

tear+pour

Start by tearing up ¼ **of a baguette** and adding it to a large bowl. Measure out ½ **cup of extra virgin cold-pressed olive oil** and **1 to 2 tablespoons of vinegar** and add to the bowl so that the bread starts to soak up the liquid.

slice+season

Have kids chop **8 tomatoes** and add to the bowl with the bread. Using a garlic press, add **1 garlic clove** to the bowl. Season with **2 teaspoons of sugar** and **3 teaspoons of salt.**

blend+chill

Pour the bread and tomato mixture into a blender and turn on high speed until thick and creamy. Taste the gazpacho and add more **salt** and/or **sugar to taste.** Put in the fridge and let chill for at least one hour—and up to 24 hours.

chop+mix

Have kids chop up **2 small cucumbers** and tear up **2 tablespoons of fresh tarragon** and add to a medium bowl. Add **1 cup of corn.** Toss together with a drizzle of olive oil and a pinch of salt and serve on top of the gazpacho. Enjoy with *Cheesy Herb Flatbread!*

¡BUEN PROVECHO!

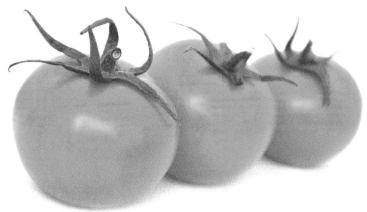

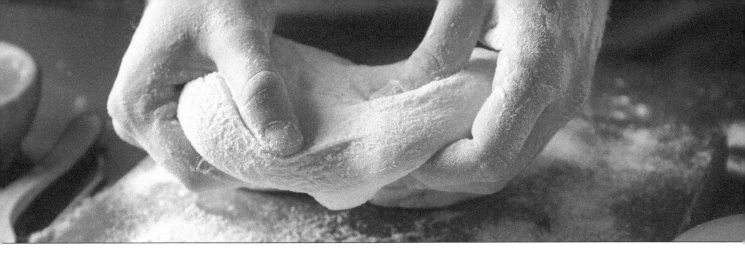

cheesey herby flatbread

ingredients

4 C all-purpose flour
1 tsp baking powder
1 tsp salt

2 C plain yogurt
1½ C Monterrey Jack cheese
fresh and/or dried herbs
olive oil

mix+knead+roll+nap

Have kids mix together **4 cups of flour**, **1 teaspoon of baking powder,** and **1 teaspoon of salt** into a large bowl. Stir in **2 cups of yogurt** until the dough is too stiff for a spoon, then knead it in the bowl until it holds together well, adding more flour if necessary. Have kids chop up or grate 1½ **cups of cheese** and add to the dough. Turn dough out on a floured surface and cut into pieces for flatbread. Have kids continue kneading their dough for about 5 minutes until the dough feels smooth and elastic. Have them add any **fresh and/or dried herbs** to the dough as they wish. Roll the dough into balls and put the dough balls in an oiled bowl, covered with a damp and clean dishtowel, and set aside to rest (nap!) at room temperature.

press+puff

After at least a 30 to 60 minute dough-ball nap, coat each dough ball in olive oil. Then give each child a dough ball and have them press the dough flat into round discs. One piece of dough should be less than a ¼ inch thick. The thinner the dough, the better! Now brush some **olive oil** on a hot skillet on your stove. Lay the dough on the hot griddle and cook it over a medium heat for 2 to 3 minutes. It will puff up in places or all over, and there may be some blackish-brown spots on the bottom. Totally OK! Slide a spatula under the flatbread and flip it, then let the flatbread cook for a minute or two, just until it finishes puffing up into a balloon and begins to color lightly on top. Fit as many bread disks as you can on your skillet. You can even try to barbecue the flatbread!

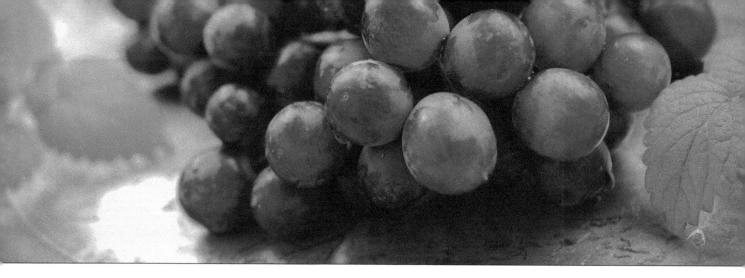

easy grape granizados

ingredients

2 C organic green seedless grapes

4 T sugar

3 to 4 fresh mint leaves

1 fresh lime

measure+squeeze+blend

Have kids measure out **2 cups of grapes**, 2 tablespoons of water, **4 tablespoons of sugar**, and **1 to 2 mint leaves** and add to your blender. Squeeze the juice from **1 fresh lime** and pour into the blender with the grapes. Add the lid and blend, blend, blend until smooth.

freeze+stir+scrape

Pour the grape mixture into a shallow baking pan and POP into your freezer. Freeze until the granita mixture is frozen, stirring edges into center every 20 to 30 minutes, for about 1½ hours. Using a fork, scrape granita into flaky crystals. Cover tightly and freeze again.

garnish+serve

Scrape granita into bowls. Garnish with **extra grapes and mint leaves.** Serve and ENJOY!

Can be made 1 day ahead and kept frozen.

Time for a Laugh!

Why did the tomato blush?

Because he saw the salad dressing!

thyme for a fun activity

Herbaceous Homemade Playdough

Playdough is a great way to incorporate creativity and sensory play into your child's day, and it's even better when it smells OH-SO-GOOD! Try this recipe the next time you have leftover herbs.

Ingredients:

1 cup warm water
2 cups all-purpose flour
½ cup salt
2 teaspoons oil (vegetable oil or olive oil will work!)
chopped fresh herbs of your choice
(rosemary, thyme, basil, etc.)

Supplies:

large saucepan or pot
stovetop
food coloring
large spoon
cutting board

Directions

- **Select the herb(s) you would like your playdough to smell like.** Herbs with a strong aroma like rosemary, mint, basil, etc. work great! Chop your fresh herbs into tiny pieces and set aside.

- **Pour 1 cup of warm water into a small bowl** and add a few drops of your **favorite food coloring,** giving that a quick stir. Set the water aside.

- **On your stovetop in a large saucepan or pot, add the dry ingredients:** 2 cups of flour and ½ cup of salt.

- **Pour in the colored water and 2 teaspoons of oil.**

- **Stir everything together** with a large spoon and cook on **medium heat** for about 3 minutes until it forms a ball.

- **Remove from the heat** and carefully turn the ball onto the cutting board. Let it cool before handling.

- **Add your chopped herbs** into the dough and knead for several minutes until the dough is springy and smooth. Give it a smell — does it need more herbs?

- **Store in an airtight container** or resealable plastic bag in the refrigerator for up to 3 months.

FALL

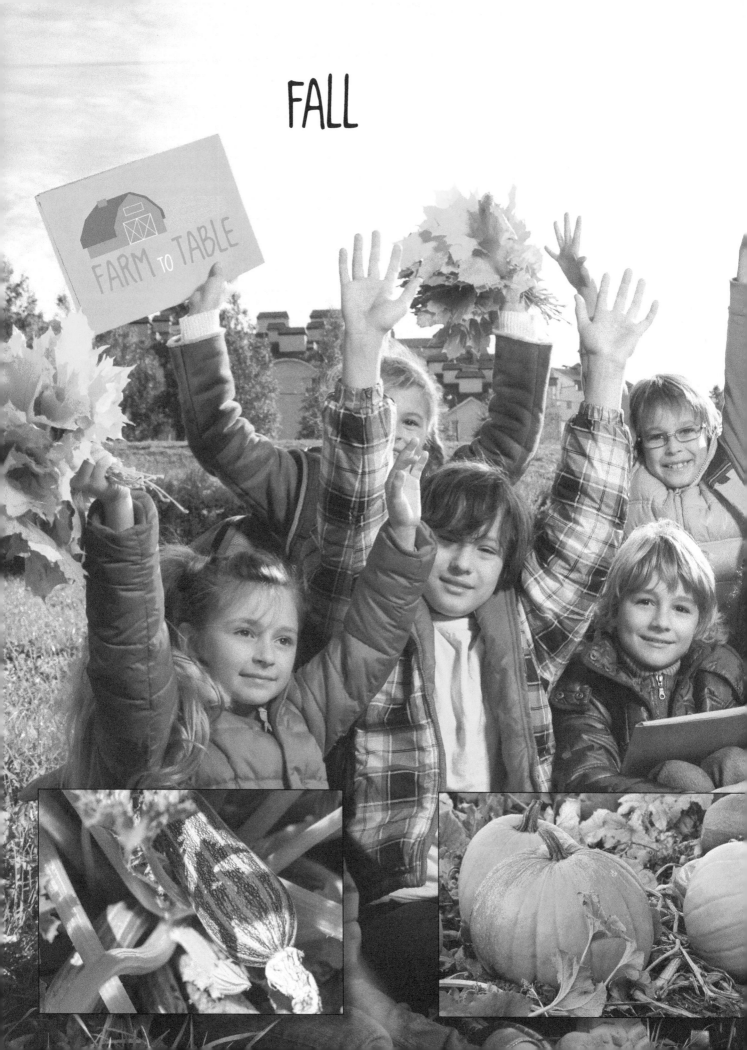

Oh, Autumn, how lovely it is to see you again! When the warm months turn chilly, we get to enjoy the luxury of decadent sandwiches, hearty plates of pasta, pumpkin pancakes, and steaming cups of hot tea to keep us warm and energized. This is the season for thanks. We are incredibly thankful for farmers in the harvest season who provide us with nourishing, delicious foods that are key components in these fun and unique fall recipes to enjoy with your friends and family.

"It's the first day of autumn! A time of hot chocolatey mornings, and toasty marshmallow evenings, and, best of all, leaping into leaves! - *Winnie the Pooh*

"If a year was tucked inside of a clock, then autumn would be the magic hour." - *Victoria Erickson*

Laugh Time: What does the farmer always wear in the fall? A harVEST!

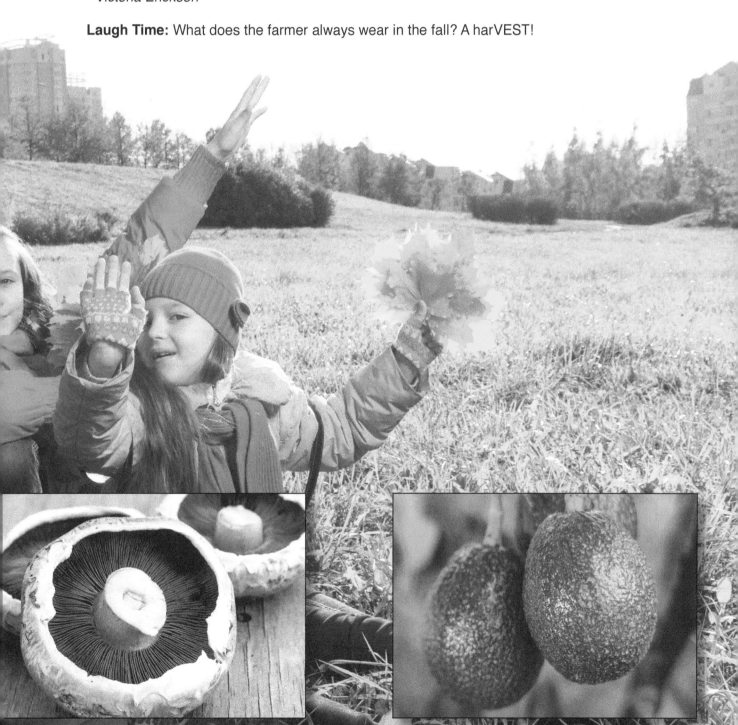

Autumn Avocado Street Tacos + Harvest Mexican Slaw + Cilantro Crema + Melon Agua Fresca

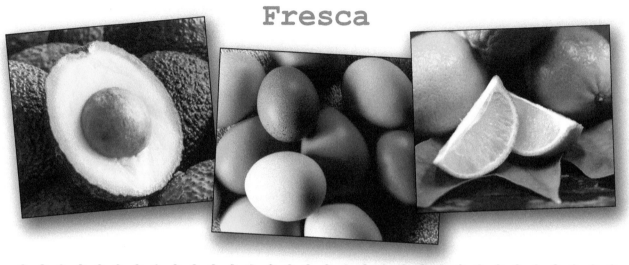

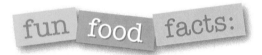

The history of Tacos

In Mexico, the word taco is a generic term like the English word sandwich. A taco is simply a tortilla wrapped around a filling. The filling can consist of practically any ingredient and be prepared in a number of different ways, though tacos are generally made with soft or fried corn tortillas. Often, the geographic region determines the contents of a taco, and people eat tacos as an entree or a snack.

The exact origin of tacos is not entirely known. However, it is believed the taco originated in the 19th century in Mexican silver mines because the first type of taco was known as *tacos de minero,* meaning "miner's tacos."

The taquería (taco shop) plays an important role in the history of tacos. For many years, women migrants sold tacos in Mexico City, creating a hub for people to sample different variations of the dish. This is how street tacos came to be. Then, in the early 1900s, migrants brought the taco to the US. and the popularity of the dish began to spread throughout the country.

The featured ingredient: Avocados!

★ **Avocados are one of the only fruits to contain fat — a special kind that is really good for you!** They are also a good source of vitamin E, vitamin B6, and dietary fiber.

★ **Avocados are technically a fruit, but people eat them like a vegetable.**

★ **Avocados grow on big evergreen trees** that have a beautiful crown of smooth, glossy, dark green leaves which shade the avocados from the sun. Avocados mature slowly and steadily on the tree, but don't ripen until they've been picked. One tree can produce 150-500 avocados per year.

★ **Avocados come in different shapes, from oval to pear, depending on the variety.** The skin looks like fine leather and helps the fruit withstand harsh sunlight. Some avocados have a smoother skin while others have a rougher, more pebbled appearance. Most are glossy green, but a few varieties do turn purplish-black when ripe. Regardless of the exterior, all have a large inedible seed surrounded by soft, buttery, creamy-white to greenish-yellow flesh on the inside, and a delicate, nutty taste!

★ **Avocados are called "Alligator Pears"** due to their pear-like shape and green skin.

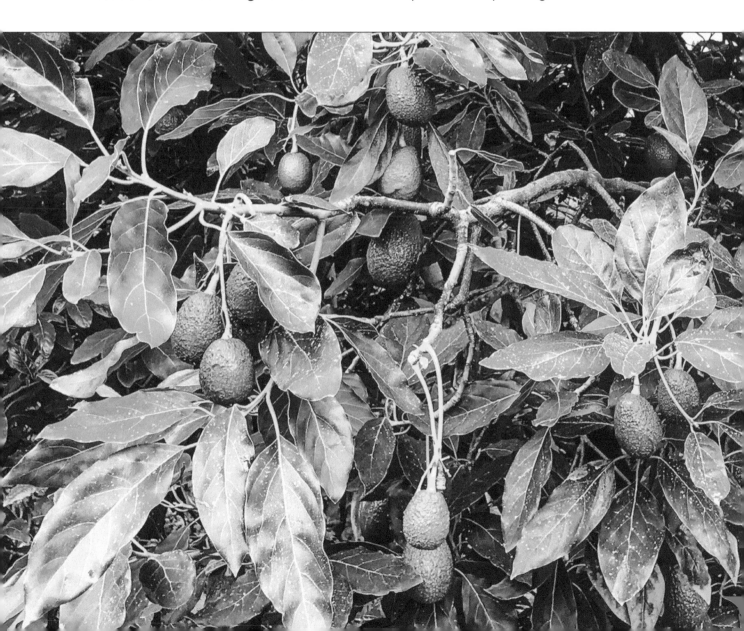

autumn avocado street tacos

ingredients

2 ripe, firm avocados

1 to 2 large eggs

½ C all-purpose flour

½ C Panko breadcrumbs

¼ C oil, for frying

8 to 12 small corn tortillas

hot sauce (optional)

cut+twist+slice

Cut around the lengthwise circumference of **2 avocados.** Twist open and remove the pit. Slice each avocado half into four to six lengthwise slices and remove the skin, leaving the flesh behind in long strips.

crack+measure

Arrange three bowls. In the first bowl, crack and whisk up **1 to 2 eggs.** In the second, measure ½ **cup of flour.** In the third, measure ½ **cup of panko breadcrumbs.**

dredge

Have your kids dip each piece of avocado first into the flour and completely cover, shaking off any excess. Then dip it into the egg and make sure it is completely coated. Last, dip it into the breadcrumbs and coat thoroughly. Set aside on a plate and continue until all the slices are done.

heat+fry

Adults, heat ¼ **cup of oil** in a skillet on your stovetop over medium-high. With a slotted spoon, gently place half of the avocado slices into the hot oil and cook for a couple minutes on the first side. Carefully turn the avocado slices over and cook a couple more minutes, until they are an even golden brown. Using a slotted spoon or tongs, transfer the avocado slices to paper towels to drain. Make the *Cilantro Crema* (see recipe on page 85).

warm+top

Warm **8 to 12 corn tortillas** on each side in a pan over your stove top, until soft. Fill each tortilla with slaw, cilantro crema, and 1 to 2 fried avocado slices on top. Top with **hot sauce,** if using!

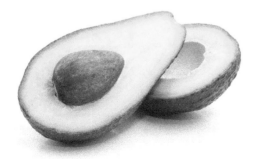
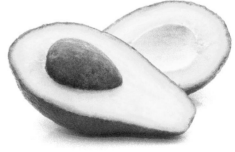

harvest mexican slaw

ingredients

¼ to ½ head red or green cabbage
1 carrot
2 radishes
2 tsp oil

2 pinches salt
2 pinches sugar
1 lime

chop+grate+slice

Finely chop **¼ to ½ head of cabbage,** grate **1 carrot,** and slice **2 radishes.** Combine in a bowl.

measure+squeeze+toss

Measure and combine **2 teaspoons of oil, 2 large pinches of salt,** and **2 large pinches of sugar.** Pour over the slaw vegetables. Squeeze the juice of **1 lime** over the slaw and toss well. Taste before serving and add any needed salt, sugar, or lime juice!

cilantro crema

ingredients

handful cilantro
1 lime
¼ C Greek yogurt or sour cream

¼ to ½ tsp salt
pinch black pepper

tear+combine

Have your kids tear up **a handful of fresh cilantro** and add to a bowl with the **juice of 1 lime,** **¼ cup of Greek yogurt or sour cream, ¼ to ½ teaspoon of salt,** and **a pinch of black pepper.**

mash+enjoy!

Mash everything together until combined and creamy. Enjoy with your tacos!

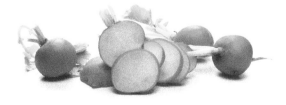

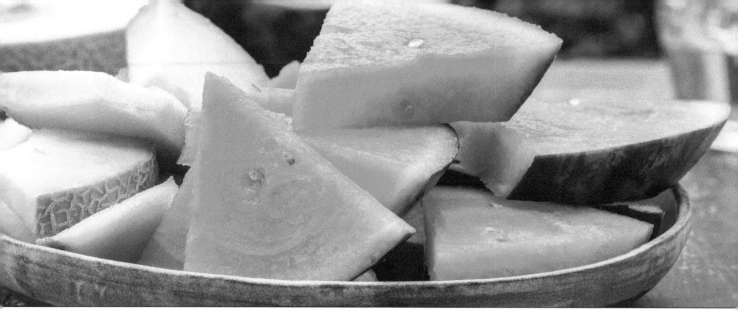

melon agua fresca

ingredients

1 lime

2 C cantaloupe, watermelon, or honeydew

½ C sugar/honey/agave

1½ C water or sparkling water

2 C ice

juice+chop

Squeeze the juice of **1 lime** into your blender or pitcher for use with an immersion blender. Chop and add **2 cups of cantaloupe, watermelon, or honeydew**. Add ½ **cup of sugar/honey/ agave** and 1½ **cups of water** or **sparkling water**.

blend+adjust

Blend until smooth and adjust flavors until just right! Serve in cups over **ice.**

Let's Finish with a Laugh!

What did the grumpy taco say to the chip?
I don't want to taco about it. It's nacho problem.

What did the Sticky Fingers Chef say to the taco?
Avocado (I've got a) crush on you!

Great Grecian Zucchini Dill Fritters
+ Herb Feta Salad + Tzatziki Dipping Sauce + Honey Yogurt Smoothies

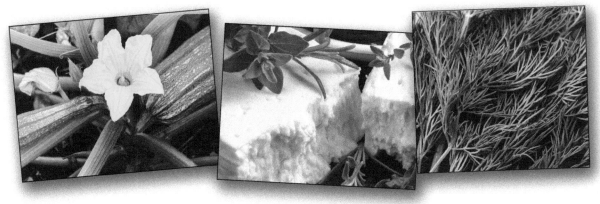

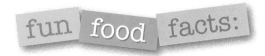

fun food facts:

Greek Food History

If we were to time-travel back to ancient Greece, it would not be difficult to find a great meal. Ancient Greeks enjoyed a wide variety of delicious and nutritious dishes, many of which we still eat to this day! Due to Greece's mild climate, farmers were able to harvest and eat a plethora of vegetables, the most common being cucumbers, fennel, celery, asparagus, and chickpeas. The Greeks also ate certain plants like dandelions (which they ate boiled), iris bulbs, and even stinging nettles!

Fruits and nuts made up a large portion of their diet, too. Wild apples, pears, and mulberries were available throughout most of Greece, as well as a fruit related to the plum called damsons. Damsons have dark blue skin and juicy flesh, and are usually eaten cooked because of their tart flavor.

None of these foods is as important to the Greeks, both ancient and modern, as the olive. The olive plays a large role not only in culinary arts but in Greek culture as well. Oil extracted from the fruit was used to light lamps, and women rubbed the oil into their skin as part of their beauty routine. According to Greek mythology, Athena, goddess of wisdom, gifted the olive tree to the people of Athens for its rich foliage and abundance of fruit. To this day, the olive branch is an important symbol representing friendship and peace.

The way that Greeks ate was also significant. Having a meal was not only about eating food; it was also a chance to talk and enjoy the company of family and friends. A Greek meal was an event! This is still the case in modern-day Greece, where dinner with friends and family may last for hours!

The featured ingredient: Zucchinis!

★ **Zucchini, or Cucurbita pepo, is a member of the cucumber and melon family.**

★ **Inhabitants of Central and South America have been eating zucchini for several thousand years,** but the zucchini we know today is a variety of summer squash developed in Italy. Though zucchinis have been grown in Italy for hundreds of years they only became popular in the US in the 1950s.

★ **The word zucchini comes from an Italian word for "small (baby) squash."** The word squash comes from the Native American *skutasquash*, or "green thing eaten green."

★ **Zucchinis are a source of potassium, vitamin A, and vitamin C.**

★ **Today, zucchini is a favorite of home gardeners.** There have been several zucchinis weighing in at over thirteen pounds!

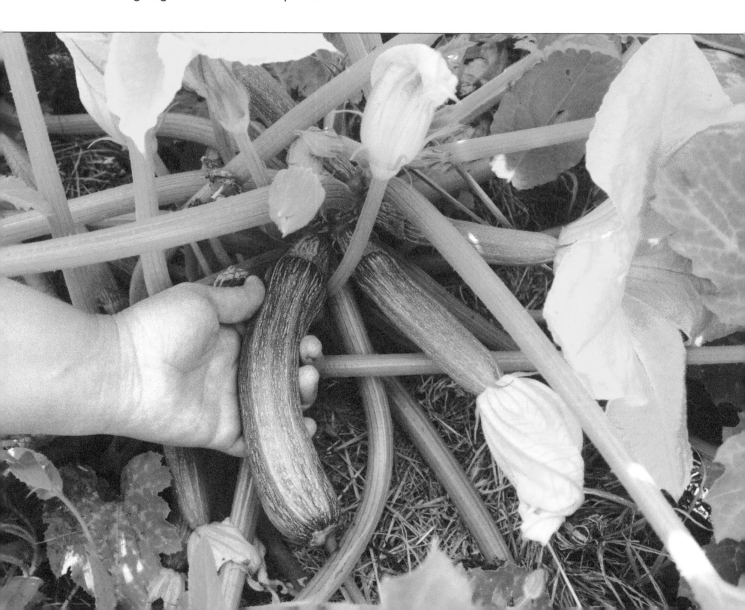

great grecian zucchini dill fritters

ingredients

2 medium zucchinis (2 C grated)

half bunch fresh dill

1 egg

½ tsp sea salt (+ more to taste)

big pinch dried oregano

¼ C all-purpose flour

2 T feta cheese

olive oil (for cooking)

grate+chop+squeeze

Have kids grate **2 cups of zucchini.** Chop **half a bunch of dill** into small bits. Now squeeze out as much of the moisture as possible from the zucchini. You can put the vegetables in a clean dish towel or use clean hands to squeeze the juice out (this will ensure your fritters hold together while cooking). Have kids combine zucchini and dill in a large bowl.

crack+mix+brown

Pre-heat your oven to 300 degrees F. Crack and mix in **1 egg, ½ teaspoon of salt,** and a **BIG pinch of dried oregano.** Add **¼ cup of flour** to the bowl and stir to blend well. Finally, stir in **2 tablespoons of feta cheese.** Heat a large drizzle of **olive oil** in your skillet over medium heat. Using about 2 tablespoons of the zucchini mixture for each fritter, roll mixture into small balls (add a little more flour if too sticky). Using a spatula, flatten each fritter a bit after placing in the skillet and cook until brown and cooked through, about 3 to 4 minutes per side. Sprinkle with a little salt and keep the fritters warm in the oven. Repeat with remaining zucchini mixture. Serve with the *Tzatziki Dipping Sauce and Herb Feta Salad!*

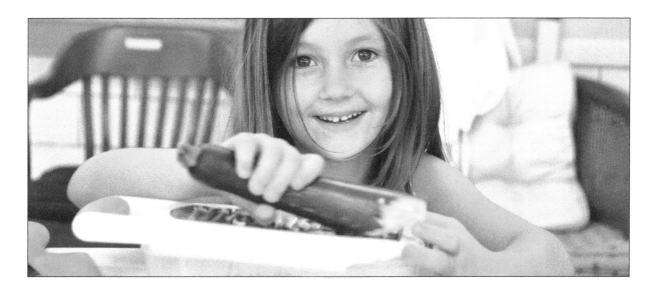

herb feta salad

ingredients

2 C fresh Italian parsley

2 T fresh dill

2 T fresh lemon juice

4 T extra virgin olive oil

2 tsp honey

½ tsp salt

pinch dried oregano

¼ C feta cheese

wash+dry+pinch

Have kids wash and dry **2 cups of parsley** and **2 tablespoons of dill.** Pick the parsley and dill leaves off the stems and pinch leaves into smaller bits, setting aside. Discard the stems.

measure+whisk

In a large bowl, have kids whisk together **2 tablespoons of lemon juice, 4 tablespoons of olive oil, 2 teaspoons of honey, ½ teaspoon of salt,** and **a pinch of dried oregano.**

toss+sit+eat

Add the parsley and dill to the bowl and toss to combine. Allow the salad to sit for at least 30 minutes in the refrigerator before serving so that flavors meld together nicely. Top with **1/4 cup of feta cheese** right before serving!

tzatziki dipping sauce

ingredients

1 small cucumber

1 small carrot

¾ C plain Greek yogurt

2 T fresh lemon juice

2 T fresh parsley, chopped

1 T fresh dill, chopped

¼ tsp sea salt (+ more to taste)

pinch dried oregano

pepper to taste

olive oil, for drizzling

grate+squeeze

Grate **1 cucumber** and **1 carrot.** Squeeze out all of the excess moisture from the vegetables.

measure+mash+season

Measure out ¾ **cup of yogurt, 2 tablespoons of lemon juice, 2 tablespoons of parsley, 1 tablespoon of dill, ¼ teaspoon of salt, a pinch of oregano,** and **pepper to taste** and add to a bowl with the cucumber and carrot. Mash with a whisk or spoon. Taste and adjust seasoning to your liking, adding more salt, pepper, and/or lemon juice, if necessary. Finish with a drizzle of **olive oil** on top!

● ●

honey yogurt smoothie

ingredients

2 bananas
1 C yogurt
2 tsp vanilla extract

1 T honey
2 C ice

peel+plop

Have kids peel **2 bananas** and plop them into the blender.

add+blend

Have kids measure **1 cup of yogurt, 2 teaspoons of vanilla extract, 1 tablespoon of honey,** and **2 cups of ice.** Blend until creamy and thick!

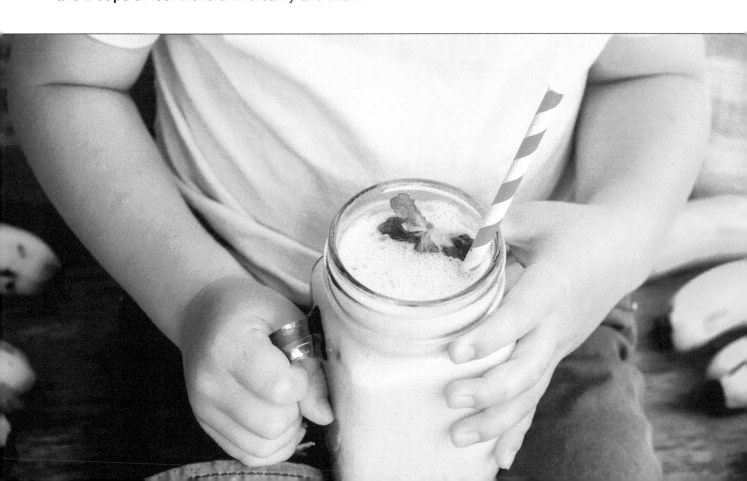

thyme for a fun activity

A Time for Gathering and Gaming

Autumn has traditionally been a time for families and communities to gather and celebrate a fruitful harvest. **The next time your family gathers at the dinner table, give these quick and easy games a try!**

Surprise Story

🚜 **One person starts off a story with a made-up sentence,** and then each person adds a sentence of their own. Who knows where the story will take you!?

🚜 **To play a different version,** each person makes up a story one word at a time!

Something's Missing

🚜 **One person takes something from the table and hides it in their lap** while everyone else has their eyes closed. When everyone opens their eyes, you have to guess what's missing!

The Farmer's Cat

🚜 **Everyone goes around the table** to describe the farmer's cat using an adjective in this sentence: "The farmer's cat is a (blank) cat."

🚜 **Start with the letter "A,"** everyone describing the cat with a different "A" adjective. For example, one person might say "The farmer's cat is an active cat" and the next person could say "The farmer's cat is an angelic cat."

🚜 **When everyone has finished the first** letter, travel through the rest of the alphabet.

🚜 **For a shortened version of the game,** say only one sentence total for each of the letters of the alphabet.

Let's Finish with a Laugh!

What kind of vegetable likes to look at animals?
A zoo-chini!

What do you call a nervous zucchini?
An edgy veggie.

Hearty Italian Lentil Bolognese Pasta + Tasty Tricolore Radicchio Salad + Outrageous Orange Italiano Ice

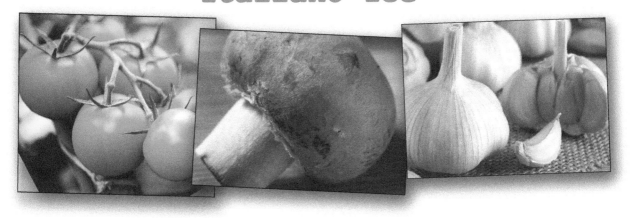

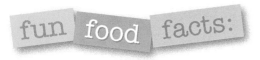

fun food facts:

Lucky Lentils!

In many parts of the world, January 1 is an opportunity to start a new year with new hopes and dreams. New Year's food traditions vary from culture to culture, but there can be so many similarities. Lentils are beloved across the globe. Lentils guarantee full and happy bellies and some say they create delicious luck to start the new year off right! In some cultures, lentils are symbolic of money. Their small, round shape makes them look like coins.

In Italy, it is tradition to eat *cotechino con lenticchie* or lentils with sausages, just after midnight— for luck and abundance in the new year. Germans also eat lentils and pork, in the form of *Eintopf* which means "One pot" lentil soup with sausages. In Brazil, the first meal of the New Year is also lentil soup or lentils and rice, and in Japan, the *osechi-ryori,* a group of symbolic dishes eaten at the new year includes lentils and sweet black beans … all for good luck, good health, and the hope of growing rich!

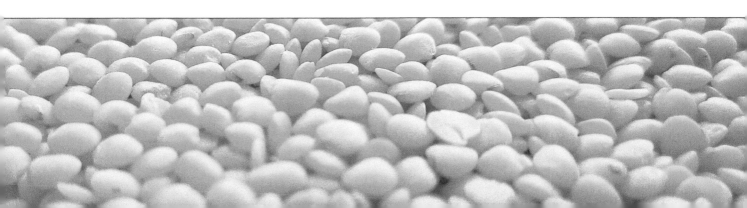

- ★ **Legumes are the flowering plants of the pea family.** The pods (they are really fruits!) of these plants are what we eat. Some delicious legumes are lentils, peas, peanuts, beans, and soybeans.

- ★ **Humans have eaten lentils for tens of thousands of years.** Remains of lentils dated to 11,000 BCE were found in a cave in Greece!

- ★ **Lentils are usually bought dried, and they can be stored for a long time.** They're also healthy and inexpensive to buy, making them a great food source.

- ★ **Because of their small size, lentils cook much more quickly than dried beans.**

- ★ **Lentils can be eaten in many wonderfully delicious ways.** They can be eaten soaked, spouted, boiled, fried, or baked.

- ★ **Lentils are loaded with protein, fiber, folate, iron, zinc, potassium, and vitamin B6 —** all good things for your body!

- ★ **Eating lentils is good for our heart health, good for our digestion, boosts our energy, and helps keep us from getting sick.**

- ★ **More than half of the world's lentils are grown in India and Canada.** In the US, most lentils are grown in Washington, Idaho, Montana, and North Dakota.

- ★ **The word "lentil" comes from the Latin word for lens.** Eyeglass lenses were actually named after lentils! Cool!

• •

hearty italian lentil bolognese pasta

ingredients

5 green onions	1 T Italian seasoning
2 large carrots	4 C water (boiling)
2 celery stalks	1 C red lentils
2 garlic cloves	16 oz fettuccini noodles, dried or fresh
1 zucchini	28 oz can crushed tomatoes
8 oz cremini mushrooms	1 tsp salt
2 T olive oil + more for sautéing	shredded or shaved Parmesan cheese
1 T sugar	

snip+peel+grate+slice

Use a clean pair of scissors to snip **5 green onions** into small bits. Peel and grate **2 carrots** carefully using a box grater and slice **2 celery stalks**.

smash+peel+mince

Using the heel of your hand, smash **2 garlic cloves** against a cutting board (adults might need to help with this!). Then peel the garlic and mince up the cloves into small bits.

chop+sauté+season

Chop **1 zucchini** into very small bits! Chop **8 oz of cremini mushrooms** into small bits, too. Add **2 tablespoons of olive oil** to a large skillet or soup pot. Sauté the onions, garlic, carrots, and celery over medium heat until soft. Season with **1 tablespoon of sugar** and **1 tablespoon of Italian seasoning** and stir. Add the chopped mushrooms and cook until soft.

add+boil+simmer+stir

To your skillet or stockpot, add **1 cup of red lentils** and 3 cups of water. Bring to a boil, lower to a simmer, and cook until lentils are *al dente* and water has absorbed. Meanwhile, bring **4 cups of water** to a boil in a separate pot and add **16 oz of fettuccini noodles**. Boil until noodles are *al dente,* then drain and drizzle with **olive oil** to keep them from sticking! To the lentils, stir in a **28 oz can of crushed tomatoes** and **1 teaspoon of salt.** Simmer uncovered until sauce thickens, about another 5-10 minutes. Taste and season with more salt or sugar. Serve over cooked fettuccini noodles and top with **shredded or shaved Parmesan cheese!** *Mangia bene!*

● ●

tasty tricolore
radicchio salad

ingredients

1 head endive	½ tsp Italian seasoning
1 head radicchio	½ tsp salt
1 cucumber	¼ tsp black pepper
juice of ½ an orange	shredded or shaved Parmesan cheese
¼ C olive oil	(optional)

slice+chop

Slice **1 head of endive** into ribbons. Chop **1 head of radicchio** into rough 1-inch pieces. Chop **1 cucumber** into half-moons or half-inch chunks. Add all chopped veggies to a mixing bowl.

squeeze+whisk+toss

Squeeze the juice from ½ **an orange** into a bowl. Whisk in ¼ **cup of olive oil, ½ teaspoon of Italian seasoning, ½ teaspoon of salt,** and ¼ **teaspoon of black pepper.** Pour over chopped veggies and toss to combine! Top with **shredded or shaved Parmesan cheese,** if desired!

outrageous orange italiano ice

ingredients

3 ½ to 4 oranges
¼ C sugar

2 C ice

squeeze+measure+blend+pour

Squeeze the juice from **3½ to 4 oranges** into a blender. Measure and add ¼ **cup of sugar** and **2 cups of ice.** Blend until the mixture is thick and smooth, adding more fresh orange juice or water if you need to thin it out some. Pour into cups and shout *SALUTE* ("Cheers" in Italian)!

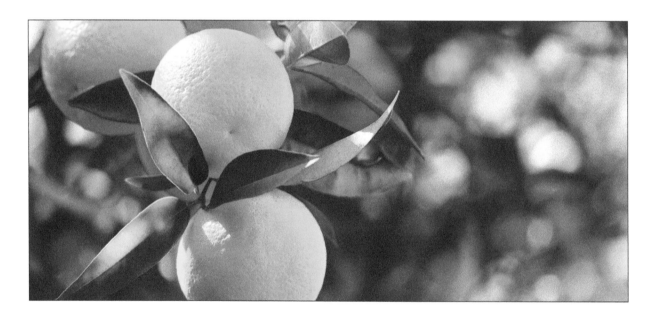

Let's Finish with a Laugh!

What does Arnold Schwarzenegger say before eating pasta?

PASTA LA VISTA, BABY.

Why did the bolognese tell the noodles to go to bed?

It was pasta bedtime!

Harvest-time Pumpkin Pie Flap-Jacks
+ Cool Cranberry Compote +
Wild Whipped Cream
in a Jar

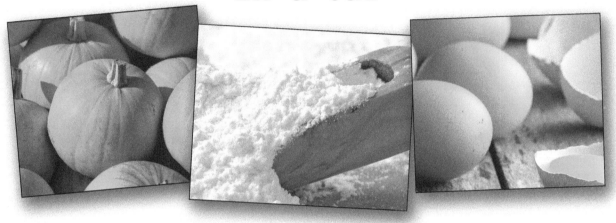

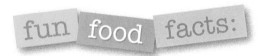

Pumpkins!

A pumpkin is really a squash?

It is! It's a member of the Cucurbita family which includes squash and cucumbers. Pumpkins are fruits!

Are pumpkins grown all over the world?

Six of the seven continents can grow pumpkins (even in Alaska)! Antarctica is the only continent that they won't grow in.

The "pumpkin capital" of the world is Morton, Illinois?

Yes, this self-proclaimed pumpkin capital is where you'll find the home of the Libby corporation's pumpkin industry.

The Irish brought this tradition of pumpkin carving to America?

The tradition originally started with the carving of turnips. When the Irish immigrated to the US, they found pumpkins a plenty and they were much easier to carve for their ancient holiday of Halloween.

- ★ **Pumpkins are 90 percent water** and contain potassium and vitamin A.
- ★ **Pumpkin flowers** are edible.
- ★ **The largest pumpkin pie ever made was over five feet in diameter and weighed over 350 pounds.** It used 80 pounds of cooked pumpkin, 36 pounds of sugar, 12 dozen eggs and took six hours to bake.
- ★ **In early colonial times,** pumpkins were used as an ingredient for the crust of pies, not the filling.
- ★ **Pumpkins were once recommended for removing freckles** and curing snake bites.
- ★ **The largest pumpkin ever grown** weighed 1,140 pounds.
- ★ **Eighty percent of the pumpkin supply** in the US is available in October.
- ★ **Native Americans flattened strips of pumpkins,** dried them, and wove them into mats. They also used pumpkin seeds for food and medicine.

harvest-time pumpkin pie flap jacks

ingredients

1 small fresh 'sugar' pie pumpkin

1 large egg

⅓ C light or dark brown sugar

1 C milk

3 T canola or vegetable oil

2 C all-purpose flour

2 tsp baking powder

2 tsp baking soda

½ tsp sea salt

2 heaping tsp ground cinnamon

1 tsp pumpkin pie spice

1 C semi-sweet chocolate chips

1 C canned pumpkin puree

cut+scoop+chop

Carefully cut open-up **1 pumpkin**. Have the kids scoop out the seeds! Ask kids to CHOP up or GRATE the fresh pumpkin flesh into very small, tiny diced up bits that measure to ½ cup of fresh diced pumpkin. Add to a bowl and set to the side.

crack+whisk

Have kids crack open **1 large egg** into a large bowl. Measure **⅓ cup of light or dark brown sugar, 1 cup of milk** and **3 tablespoons of oil** into the bowl with the egg and beat together until creamy and light yellow. This is the wet mix.

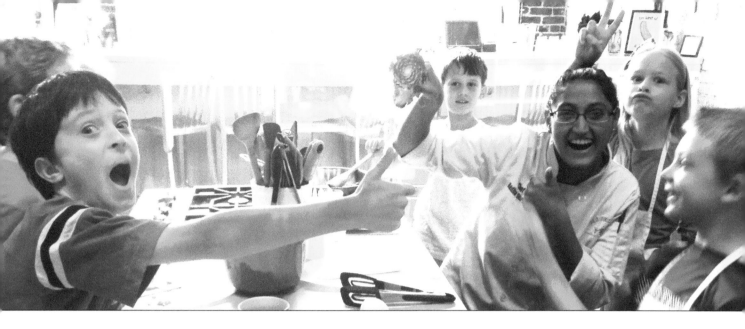

mix+measure+whisk

Have kids mix and measure: **2 cups flour, 2 teaspoons baking powder, 1 teaspoon of baking soda, ½ teaspoon of salt, 2 heaping teaspoons of cinnamon and 1 teaspoon of pumpkin pie spice** and whisk… this is the dry mix.

stir+fold

Stir the wet mix into the dry mix. Ask kids to fold in (it means to carefully mix) the ½ cup of fresh grated / diced pumpkin that you already prepared. Add **1 cup of chocolate chips** and then **1 cup of pumpkin puree.**

cook+flip+cook

Cook 1/8 cup of the batter for 2 minutes per side or until golden brown and bubbly in your pre-oiled skillet over medium heat. Flip over and cook the other side until golden brown and puffed. Make as many pancakes you can. Top with the *Cool Cranberry Compote + Wild Whipped Cream*

● ●

cool cranberry compote

ingredients

1 to 2 C fresh cranberries

½ C sugar, brown sugar, honey (or 4 to 5 packs of stevia)

pinch salt

1 lime

chop+smash+drizzle

CHOP or SMASH up **1 to 2 cups of cranberries** into little bits, drizzle ½ **cup of sugar, brown sugar, honey** on top. Add **a pinch of salt, a squeeze of lime juice**, and blend with your hand blender and set to the side. Serve with the *Harvest-time Pumpkin Pie Flap Jacks!*

wild whipped cream

ingredients

1 pint whipping cream
pinch sea salt

2 to 4 T brown sugar
1 glass or plastic jar with a tight-fitting lid

shake+whisk+SCREAM

Fill a glass or plastic jar with a tight-fitting lid ½ **full with whipping cream** and **a pinch of salt.** Have the kids shake, shake, shake, shake until it becomes thick. Whisk in **2 to 4 tablespoons of brown sugar** and eat with the pancakes. Scream: "YUMMY-IN-MY-TUMMY!"

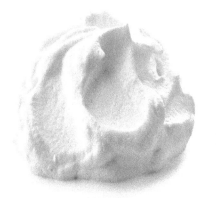 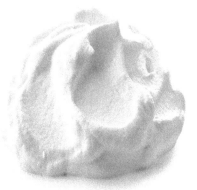 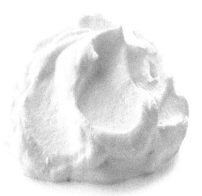

Let's Finish with a Laugh!

What did one Jack-o-lantern say to the other?
Cut it out!

What's the ratio of a pumpkin's circumference to its diameter?
Pumpkin Pi (3.14159)

What do you get when you cross a snowman and a vampire?
Frostbite!

What's black, white, orange, and waddles?
A penguin carrying a Jack-o-lantern!

Tasty Toasted
Portobello Reuben Sammies
+ Quick-Pickled Cabbage +
1,000 Isle Dressing +
Very Vanilla Shakes

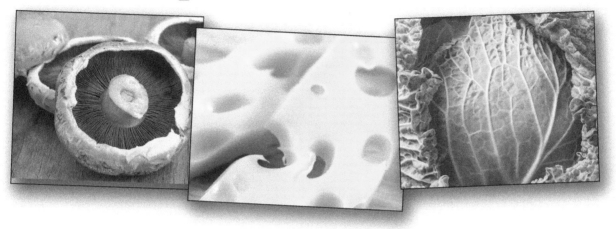

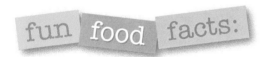

Let's learn about Mushrooms!

Portobello mushrooms are native to Italy and have been grown since ancient times.
Portobello mushrooms are the largest mushrooms you'll find in most grocery stores. Creminis are the less mature version of portobellos, which are harvested once they are fully grown!

The word *portobello* literally means "beautiful door" in Italian. The name was given to overgrown mushrooms in an attempt to sell more of them in the 1980s! Cremini mushrooms are Italian in origin while portobellos were named and marketed in the US.

Mushrooms are a kind of fungus that look like umbrellas! They grow in places like yards, forests, fields, and gardens. Many fungi eat by breaking down dead plants.

Some mushrooms are good to eat, like portobellos, while others are very poisonous.
Never eat a mushroom you find growing outside!

The Honey Mushroom in the Blue Mountains of Oregon is the world's largest living thing.
It is actually a mushroom colony and is believed to be at least 2,000 years old! It covers almost four square miles!

Even though mushrooms don't use sun for energy, they use the sun to produce vitamin D, just like humans do!

A brief history of the Reuben Sandwich!

There are many origin stories for the Reuben! Many people have claimed to be the inventors of this legendary sandwich, including a man named Reuben who owned a restaurant and said he created the sandwich one night for Charlie Chaplin's (hungry!) leading lady.

Another story says the sandwich was invented by a man named Bernard Schimmel for his friend, Reuben Kulakofsky. Both Reuben and Bernard were part of a weekly poker group at a hotel in Omaha, Nebraska called The Blackstone. The hotel eventually put the sandwich on their lunch menu, and it started to gain fame. If your best friend named a sandwich after you, what would it have on it?

● ●

tasty toasted portobello reuben sammies + quick-pickled cabbage

ingredients

quick-pickled cabbage:
½ head white/green/red cabbage
1 C white vinegar
1½ tsp salt
1 T sugar

tasty toasted portobello reuben sammies:
3 large portobello mushrooms
¼ C olive oil (+ more for cooking)
salt and black pepper
1 loaf rye bread, sliced
Swiss cheese slices

shred+measure+boil

Using a box grater or a food processor, shred **½ a head of cabbage.** You can also use pre-shredded cabbage (you'll want about 2½ to 3 cups total). Measure and add 1½ cups water, **1 cup of vinegar, 1½ teaspoons of salt,** and **1 tablespoon of sugar** to a skillet and bring to a boil. Then add shredded cabbage, stir to submerge, and turn off heat. Let cabbage sit in this brine while you make the rest of the recipes. Reserve some brine to make the 1,000 Isle Dressing.

rinse+twist+scrape+slice

Rinse loose dirt from **3 portobello mushrooms.** Twist off their stems and discard. Scrape the gills from underneath each mushroom cap and discard. Then slice mushroom caps into ½-inch slices. Add mushroom slices to a mixing bowl.

drizzle+mix+sauté

Drizzle mushroom caps with ¼ **cup of olive oil** and sprinkle with **salt** and **black pepper.** Stir to mix, then sauté over low heat until mushrooms are tender and brown in spots. Transfer sautéed mushrooms to a bowl.

drizzle+toast+melt

Drizzle skillet with more **olive oil,** then add **sliced Rye bread**. If using a toaster oven, add oilve oil *after* toasting. Layer on sautéed mushrooms and **sliced Swiss cheese.** Cover skillet and toast until cheese has melted and bread is golden brown. Then top each toast slice with *Quick-Pickled Cabbage* and let warm through. Finish by spreading ***1,000 Isle Dressing*** (recipe below) on each sandwich. Eat Sammies open-faced or closed!

1,000 isle dressing

ingredients

½ cucumber
¼ C ketchup
¼ C mayonnaise
¼ tsp garlic/onion powder

1 tsp soy sauce
pinch salt
½ orange (juice of)

shred+measure+add+whip

Shred **1 cucumber** and set aside half for the *Very Vanilla Shakes*. Add the other half to a mixing bowl. Measure and add ¼ **cup of ketchup,** ¼ **cup of mayonnaise,** ¼ **teaspoon of onion/garlic powder, 1 teaspoon of soy sauce, a pinch of salt, 2 teaspoons of** *Quick-Pickled Cabbage* **brine, juice from ½ an orange,** and ½ the shredded cucumber to the bowl. Whip with a whisk until combined, then top *Portobello Reuben Sammies* with *1,000 Isle Dressing* and ENJOY!
To make an egg-free version, substitute sour cream or coconut cream for mayonnaise.

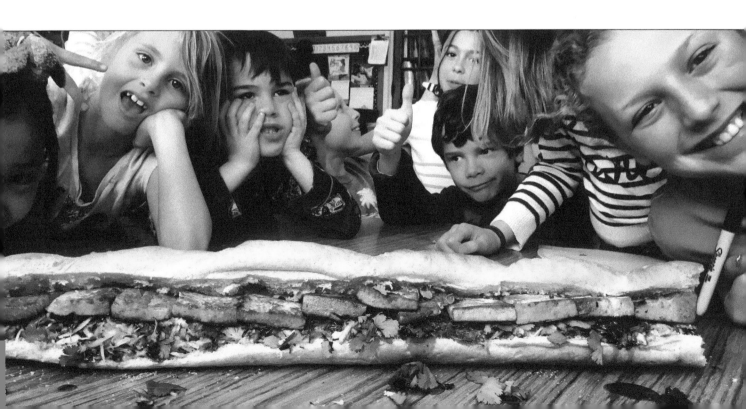

very vanilla shakes

ingredients

½ orange
1 cucumber
1½ C full-fat vanilla yogurt

1 C ice
1 tsp vanilla extract
sugar to taste

squeeze+add+blend

Squeeze juice from ½ **an orange** into a blender. Add ½ **grated cucumber** to the blender, along with **1½ cups of full-fat vanilla yogurt, 1 cup of ice,** ½ cup of water, **1 teaspoon of vanilla extract, sugar to taste.** Puree until shakes are thick and smooth, adding more water if needed to thin them out, then divide into cups and enjoy!

To make a dairy-free version, substitute 1 can of coconut milk for the yogurt.

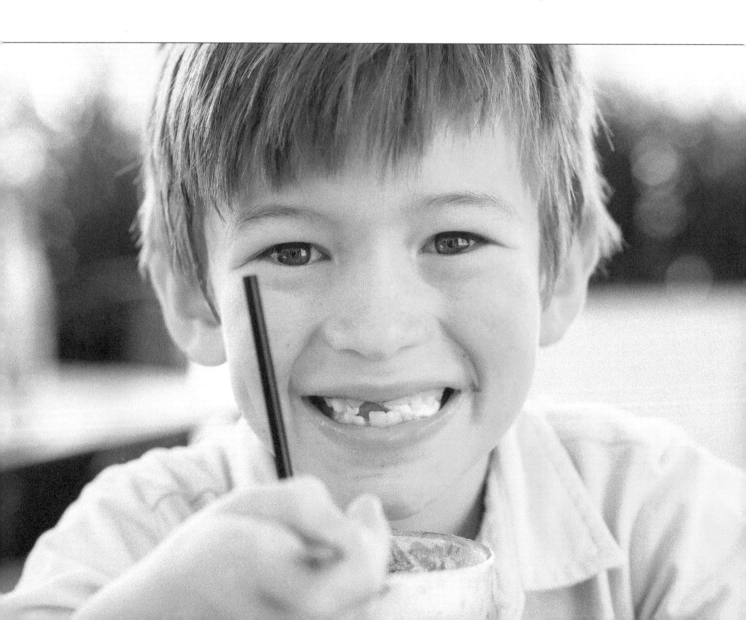

thyme for a fun activity

Hello Honey Sugar Scrub

ingredients:

¼ cup warm honey
2 tablespoons liquid coconut oil (or olive oil would work!)
½ cup brown sugar

supplies:

mixing bowl
small jar or tupperware for storage
spoon or whisk

directions

- Pour ¼ of cup warm honey into a small or medium mixing bowl. Tip: you can microwave your honey in a microwave-safe bowl or boil a small pot of water, transfer to a bowl, and set the jar of honey in the hot water to bring up the temperature.
- Add 2 tablespoons of liquid oil to the mixing bowl with the warmed honey and stir until combined.
- Sprinkle ½ cup of brown sugar into the mixing bowl and stir until all ingredients come together. At this point, you may decide you want to add more honey or sugar, depending on the consistency you like.
- Massage the scrub over your face, neck, or hands for a luxurious and all-natural exfoliation! Exfoliating removes any dead skin and lets the fresh, new skin breathe. Let it dry before rinsing off. Did you know? Honey is naturally antibacterial and full of antioxidants, which is great for your skin's well-being.
- Save any leftovers in an airtight jar.

Time for a Laugh!

Why did the Fungi leave the party?
There wasn't mushroom to dance!

Why did the Mushroom get invited to all the parties?
'Cuz he's a fungi!

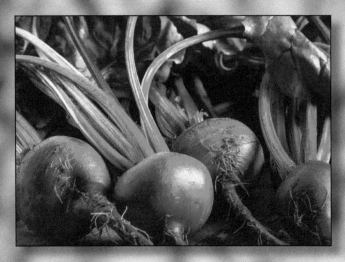

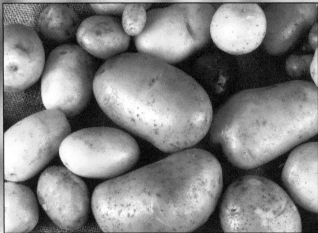

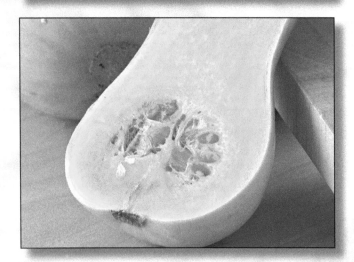

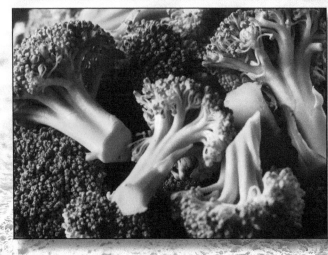

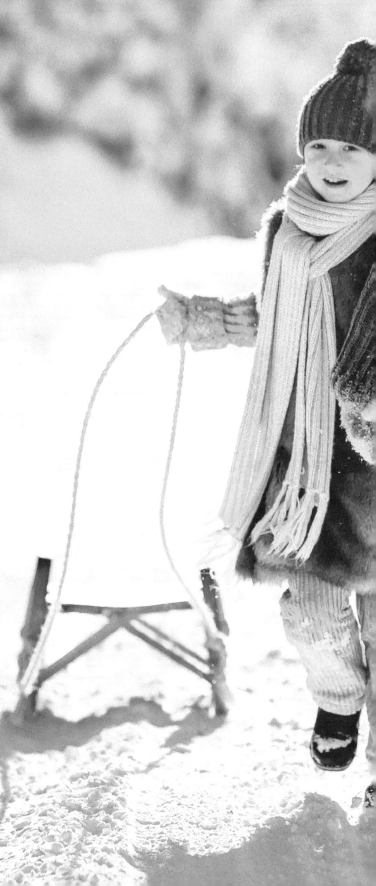

WINTER

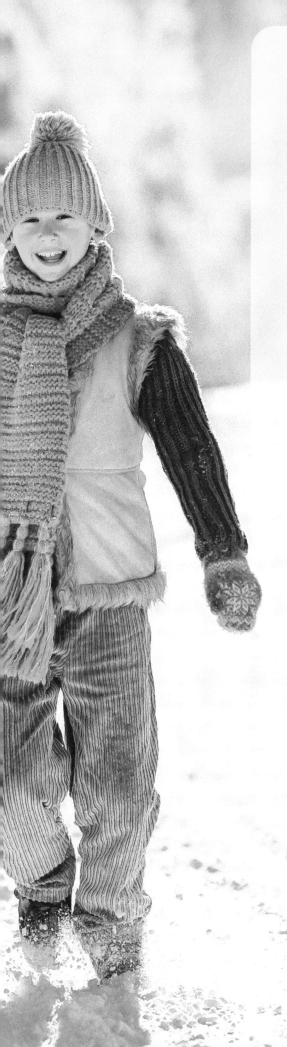

Goodness is the quiet magic of wintertime! Whither in the world you call home, winter gives us all of the cozy and snug things: favorite sweaters, winter sports, holidays, and comfort food.

When holidays with family are just around the corner, it's always good to have some hearty recipes in your back pocket. Let these winter superfood recipes embrace your family with a soul-warming bowl of butternut squash risotto, stick-to-your-ribs vegetable pot pies, and creamy broccoli bread pudding that practically bubbles over the casserole dish. It's the time of year to seek out seasonal winter produce and use it in unexpected ways, like the beets in our red velvet doughnut holes.

One kind word can warm three winter months.
- Japanese Proverb

The fire is winter's fruit. *- Arabian Proverb*

They who sing through summer must dance in the winter.
- Italian Proverb

Laugh Time: What do snowmen call their offspring?
CHILL-dren

Broccoli Bread Pudding
+ Massaged Kale Salad +
Lemon-Up 'Soda'

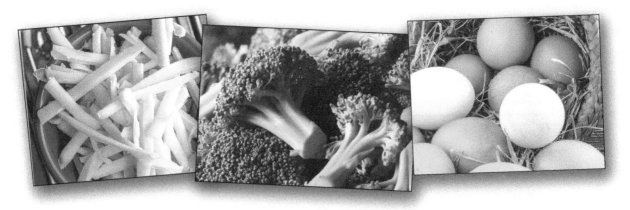

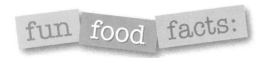

The history of Bread Pudding

Bread pudding can be traced back to the early 11th and 12th centuries. This dish was originally known as "poor man's pudding" as it was a way for the lower class to use up stale bread. Today, many people still appreciate that aspect of bread pudding, but they also love the nostalgia and simplicity of the dish. Bread pudding has solidified its reputation as a comfort food, and many restaurants have elevated this once-humble dish with unique flavors and pairings.

To make this dish, start by layering chunks of (usually) day-old bread and add a custard sauce before baking. The possibilities for the dish are endless because cooks can vary the type of bread and ingredients they add!

The featured ingredient: Broccoli!

Broccoli belongs to the brassica family and is closely related to the cabbage. Broccoli florets have a very distinct appearance — they look like small, dense trees, with greenish-white branches ending in clumps of small, rounded, and tightly packed blue-green or green flower buds. Broccoli has a delicious flavor. Unlike those wimpy summer vegetables (ha, ha), broccoli is the sweetest and best eaten during the winter months.

- **Broccoli is related to both cabbage and cauliflower** and, they are part of an important group of vegetables that can help keep your body healthy.

- **Broccoli was once known as Italian asparagus.**

- **The word Broccoli comes from the Italian word 'brocco' meaning arm or branch.**

- **One cup of raw broccoli has as much vitamin C as an orange!** Vitamin C helps keep our hearts and immune system. Don't overcook it or you'll lose some of the vitamins.

- **Broccoli also has a lot of fiber.** Think of fiber as a broom that sweeps the dirt and muck from the inside of your intestines! VER-RY important.

- **Don't underestimate the power of broccoli!** Broccoli became famous when researchers found they contained a compound called sulphoraphane, which can function as an anti-cancer agent.

- **Broccoli is also a good source of dietary fiber** and will also give you potassium, vitamin E, folate and beta carotene.

- **The first broccoli plants came from the eastern Mediterranean** and Asia Minor and spread to Italy in the 16th century.

Broccoli! So, Who are we? Here's how to find the best of us: We have beautiful, bright-green and dense clusters of tightly-closed flowerets. Our stalks and stem leaves are quite tender and yet firm. Avoid choosing any of us with yellowing flowerets and thick, woody stems!

How to Keep Broccoli: Keep us dry! We don't like being damp. Store us in a vented plastic bag in the refrigeratior for up to 5 days.

History of Broccoli: We come from the eastern Mediterranean and Asia Minor, but then we journeyed to Italy in the 16th century to eventually made it to England and America!

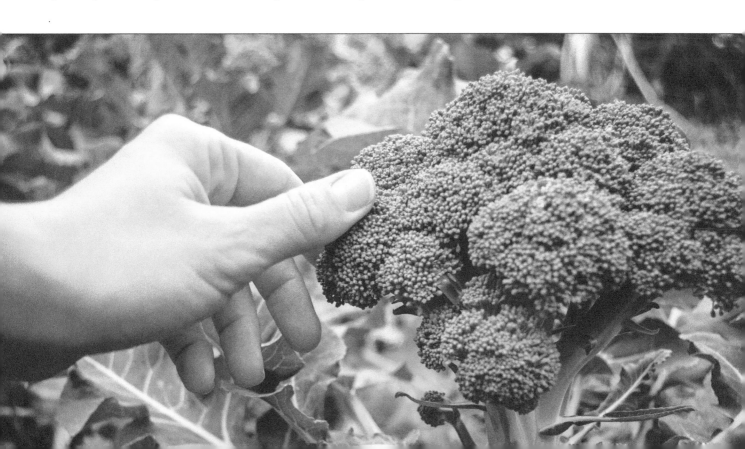

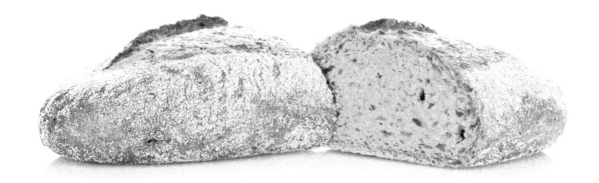

broccoli bread pudding

ingredients

½ loaf of bread
1 C Monterey Jack cheese
2 eggs
1 C milk
1 C vegetable broth
½ tsp salt + a pinch more

½ tsp dried dill
big pinch black pepper
½ lb broccoli (approx. ½ head)
oil (for cooking)

preheat+tear+grate

Preheat your oven to 350 degrees F. Tear or cut ½ **loaf of bread** into very small pieces/cubes and place in a large bowl. Grate **1 cup of cheese** and set to the side.

whisk+pour

In a medium bowl, have kids whisk together **2 eggs, 1 cup of milk, 1 cup of vegetable broth, ½ teaspoon of salt, ½ teaspoon of dill,** and **a pinch of black pepper** until well combined. Pour the mixture over the bread and let it sit.

snap+chop+sauté

Have kids snap off the tough ends of **½ lb broccoli** (approximately ½ head) and chop the tops into very small pieces. Sauté the bits of cauliflower in a little **oil** and a pinch of salt on your stovetop over medium-high heat for 3 to 5 minutes or until soft and a little browned.

fold+oil+bake

Add the cooked cauliflower to the bread mixture and fold everything together to combine the ingredients well. Add the grated cheese to the mixture and stir again. Brush some oil on the wells of your cupcake pan and fill each one about half-full with bread pudding mixture. Bake in your oven for 20 to 25 minutes or until cooked through.

massaged kale salad

ingredients

1 bunch kale
1 lemon
¼ C olive oil + more for drizzling
sea salt

2 tsp honey/agave/sugar
small handful toasted pepitas or
sunflower seeds

tear+squeeze+drizzle

In a large serving bowl, have kids tear leaves of **1 bunch of kale** (throw away the stalks) into small bits. Squeeze the juice of ½ **a lemon** over the kale along with a **drizzle of olive oil** and **sprinkle of salt.**

massage+wilt

Using clean hands, have kids massage the kale until it starts to soften and wilt, about 2 to 3 minutes. Set aside and make the dressing.

whisk+pour

Whisk together the **juice of ½ a lemon** with **2 teaspoons of honey/agave/sugar** and ¼ **cup of olive oil** until a dressing forms. Add more honey if needed. Pour the dressing over the kale and toss. Top with some **toasted pepitas or sunflower seeds,** if desired!

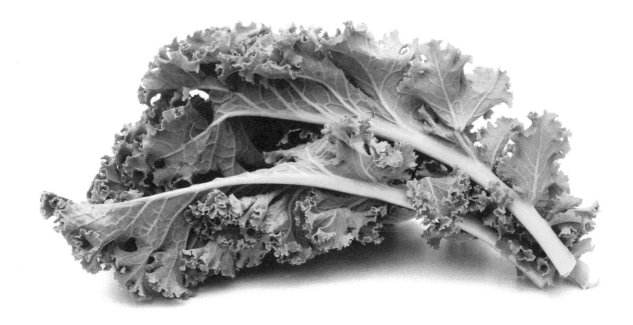

lemon-up soda

ingredients

2 lemons
½ C honey/agave/sugar

2 C ice
½ to 1 L soda water

squeeze+boil

Squeeze the **juice of 2 lemons** into a small bowl and set to the side. In a small saucepan on your stovetop, combine ½ cup of water, ½ **cup of sugar/agave/honey,** and the leftover lemon peels. Bring to a boil and cook for 2 to 3 minutes. Then turn the heat and allow to cool.

strain+discard+mix

Strain the lemon peels from the syrup and discard. Add your freshly squeezed lemon juice to the sugar syrup and mix well.

serve+top

Add 1 to 2 teaspoons of syrup to the bottom of each cup and top with **ice** and **soda water.** Enjoy!

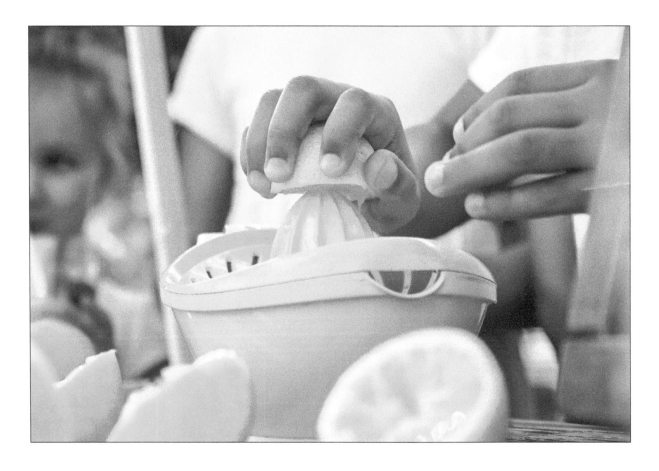

thyme for a fun activity

Mind your P's and Q's

"Minding your Ps and Qs" is a funny little phrase that dates back to the mid-1800s. Some believe the expression came from learning to handwrite the alphabet since the lower-case p and q look so similar, while others think it came from saying "please and thank you." Either way, the expression now means to "use good manners" or "be on your best behavior."

When children see adults modeling expectations, they are likely to instinctively mimic them. And ending the dinner with a sweet treat is always a fun time!

1 **Everyone at the dinner table gets 10 M&Ms** (or small candy of your choice). Your kids may be tempted to eat them, but not just yet!

2 **Share the following "game rules" or feel free to make up your own!** Throughout the course of dinner, try to catch any family member not following the rules. Anyone who lapses in table manners must give one piece of candy to the person who caught them.

3 **By the time dinner is over, the person with the most candies wins!** Enjoy a sweet treat to the end of a delicious and fun family meal.

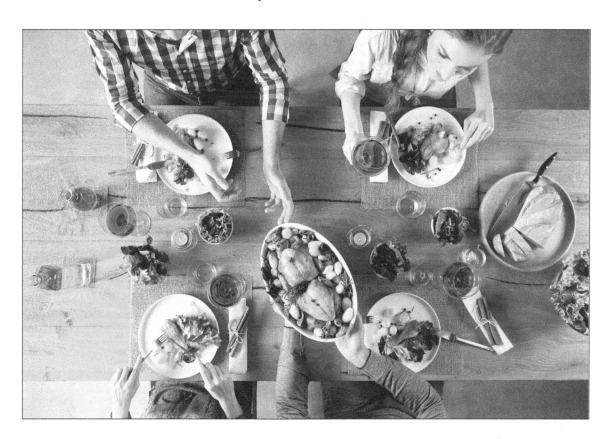

Very Veggie Pot Pie Cups
+ 'Caramel' Apple Shazam Shakes

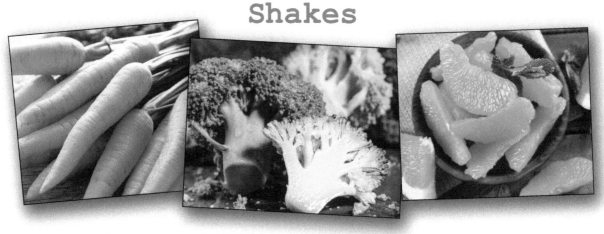

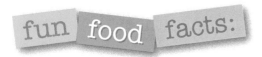

The history of Pot Pies!

Much like the oral tradition of storytelling where details tend to change from generation to generation, the pot pie has undergone a number of changes overtime. Although historians debate the exact origin of this dish, it is known that ancient Romans served pastries stuffed with meats and vegetables, often at feasts. Stuffed pies came back into fashion during the Middle Ages when crafting pies for royalty became an art form. Commoners also ate this dish when they discovered it could feed more mouths when bread was added to the filling.

American settlers traveling west were also known to bring pot pie variations with them. Many different cultures all over the world put their own, unique spin on this dish. The combination of all these cultures in North America eventually resulted in dessert pies.

Is pot pie good for you? Pot pie covers most of the food groups, except fruit, but its healtfulness really depends on your chosen recipe. If you load it with salt and only meat, it is less healthy, but if you add lots of veggies, like our Sticky Fingers Cooking *Very Veggie Pot Pie Cups*, it can be much healthier!

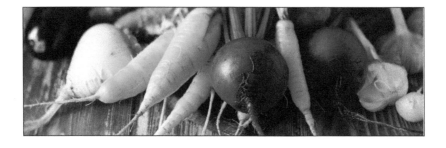

The featured ingredient: Vegetables!

★ **If you want to get the most vitamins and nutrients out of your vegetables, try eating the skins when you can!** Vegetable skins and the layer directly underneath hold the most nutritional content.

★ **Vegetables are plants that are grown for food purposes** and usually include the stem, and/or root.

★ **You can cook vegetables in a number of ways,** including baking, roasting, steaming, blanching, boiling, frying, grilling, and marinating, which can result in different textures, flavors, and nutritional value.

★ **Vegetables are generally healthier for you than fruit.** While root vegetables are higher in natural sugars, vegetables as a whole are lower in sugar and higher in fiber than most fruits and are more densely packed with nutrients.

★ **Broccoli and bell peppers are the vegetables with the most vitamin C.** Broccoli contains just as much calcium as a glass of milk and actually more vitamin C than oranges. Green bell peppers have double the amount of the vitamin C when compared to oranges, and red/yellow/orange bell peppers have quadruple that amount!

★ **Frozen vegetables are just as beneficial to our health as fresh vegetables,** though canned vegetables often contain extra sodium and may lose nutrients during the canning process.

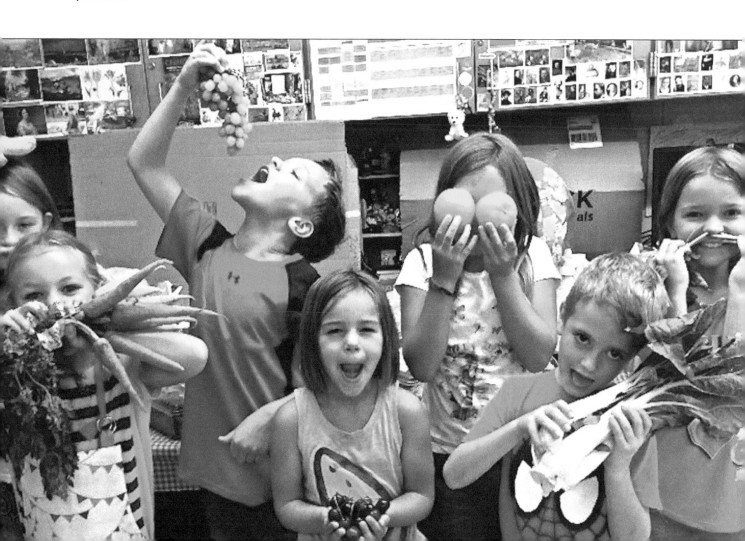

homemade pie crust

ingredients

1 stick (½ C) frozen unsalted butter   ice water

1 C + 2 T all-purpose flour

cut+rub

Have your kids cut 1 stick **(½ cup) of unsalted butter** into small cubes or slices and add to **1 cup + 2 tablespoons of flour.** Using a pastry blender or fork, cut the mixture until it resembles coarse meal. Then, have your kids use their hands to quickly rub the mixture together, so that the butter is absorbed into the flour.

drizzle+mix+roll

Gradually drizzle **ice water** into the bowl, mixing with the pastry blender or fork until the dough just comes together. Quickly shape the dough into a ball and flatten into a disk. Place on a floured surface and roll out to 1/8-inch thick. Have your kids make roundish shapes for a total of about 12 dough rounds.

very veggie pot pie cups

ingredients

1 to 2 green onions

1 garlic clove

vegetable oil or butter (for cooking)

vegetables of choice (selected from following list)

1 tsp poultry seasoning

1 tsp black pepper

1 vegetable bouillon cube

1 T cornstarch

½ C shredded cheese

preheat+chop+sauté

Preheat your oven to 400 degrees F and grease or spray a muffin pan with oil or butter. Chop **1 to 2 green onions** and **1 garlic clove** and sauté for 3 to 5 minutes in a little **vegetable oil** on your stovetop over medium heat. Meanwhile, have your kids chop, dice, slice, and/or grate their **vegetables of choice** (see following page for suggestions) into pieces that are approximately the same size.

Have fun selecting (at least!) 4 of these fresh and tasty vegetables for your pot pies:

1 zucchini

1 yellow squash

1 to 2 celery stalks

2 carrots

2 handfuls frozen green peas

2 handfuls frozen corn

2 handfuls frozen green beans

1 handful mushrooms

½ C cauliflower

½ C broccoli

1 baby eggplant

2 handfuls fresh spinach

2 handfuls fresh kale

1 bell pepper

1 tomato

1 precooked potato or sweet potato

1 handful Brussels sprouts

snip+peel+grate+slice

Add your *chopped vegetable mixture* to the skillet with the *onion and garlic*. Add **1 teaspoon of poultry seasoning**, **1 teaspoon of black pepper**, **1 vegetable bouillon cube**, and cook until vegetables are tender, approximately 5 minutes. Turn off the heat on the skillet and sprinkle on **1 tablespoon of cornstarch** and mix well. Add a little water at this point — just enough to get everything thick. Finally, add ¼ **cup of shredded cheese**. Stir to combine.

press+spoon+sprinkle

Have your kids make a mini-dough bowl with their fingers to line each cup of your mufin pan. Press the dough into the bottom and up the sides of each muffin well. Spoon the veggie mixture evenly into each cup and sprinkle with **some extra cheese**.

bake+cool

Bake for 12 to 15 minutes or until set and slightly golden. Remove from the oven and let them cool for a few minutes before removing from the muffin pan.

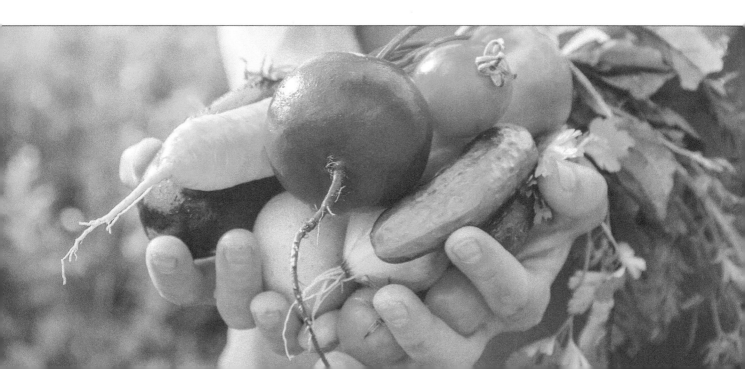

caramel apple shazam shakes

ingredients

warm water
¼ C raisins
1 to 2 apples

1 C half-and-half (or unsweetened non-dairy creamer)
pinch of salt
2 to 3 C ice

plump+chop

In a little dish, pour a little warm water over ¼ **cup of raisins** and let them sit for at least 10 minutes and up to 2 hours. Then have your kids chop **1 to 2 apples** and add them to your blender, or a pitcher for use with an immersion blender.

add+blend

Add **1 cup of half-and-half or unsweetened non-dairy creamer, a pinch of salt,** and **2 to 3 cups of ice** to your blender/pitcher and your plumped raisins. Blend and *shazam!* — you've got a delicious shake! Enjoy!

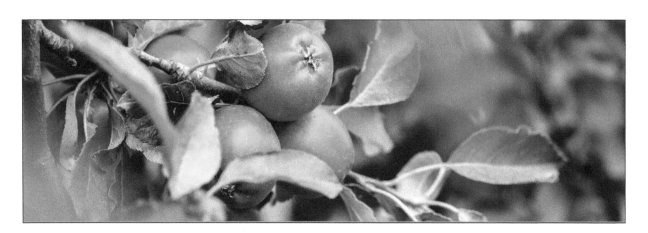

Let's Finish with a Laugh!

Why did the pot pie go to the dentist? Because
it needed a filling!

What's the best thing to put into a pot pie? Your teeth!

thyme for a fun activity

Mix, Package, Gift! DIY Spice Kits

In a small bowl, mix together all ingredients and store in an airtight container to keep fresh for months. We suggest adding sweet or savory spices to buttered popcorn!

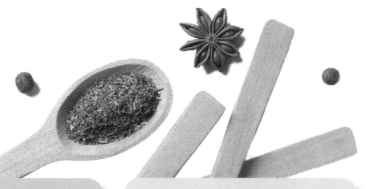

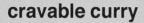

cravable curry

★ 2 tablespoons ground cumin
★ 2 tablespoons ground coriander
★ 2 teaspoons ground turmeric
★ ½ teaspoon dry mustard, ground ginger, black pepper, salt
★ 1 teaspoon onion powder
★ ¾ teaspoon garlic powder
★ ⅛ teaspoon cloves

terrific taco

★ 2 teaspoons chili powder
★ 1 ½ teaspoon paprika
★ 1 ½ teaspoon cumin
★ 1 teaspoon onion powder
★ ¾ teaspoon garlic powder
★ ½ teaspoon sea salt
★ ¼ teaspoon sugar
★ tiny pinches of cloves and cinnamon

super italian

★ 2 tablespoons chopped fresh parsley
★ 1 teaspoon dried basil
★ 1 pinch oregano
★ 1 teaspoon garlic powder
★ salt and pepper to taste

sweet spice

★ 1 ½ tablespoon cinnamon
★ 1 teaspoon ground ginger
★ 1 teaspoon ground nutmeg
★ ¾ teaspoon allspice
★ ¾ teaspoon ground cloves

Red Velvet (just BEET it) Doughnut Holes
+ Mint Dust + Red Velvet Shakes

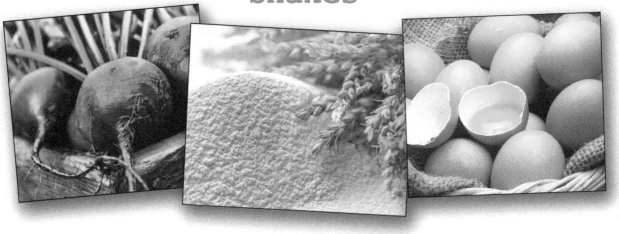

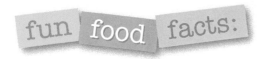

The history of Red Velvet Cake

Red Velvet Cake originated in the 1920s at New York's fancy Waldorf-Astoria Hotel. A lady had recently been in New York City on vacation and had dinner at the Waldorf-Astoria, where she ate Red Velvet cake and LOVED it! After she returned home, she wrote a letter to the hotel inquiring after the name of the chef who had invented the cake, wondering if she could have the recipe. She received the recipe in the mail in addition to a bill for $100 from the chef (adjusted for inflation, worth about $1500 today)!

The lady's attorney advised her to simply pay the bill because technically she had not asked beforehand if there would be a charge for the recipe. Angrily, she paid the bill, but had a plan up her sleeve: to "get even" with the greedy chef, every time she was on a bus or train, she would pass out 3x5-inch cards with a handwritten recipe for "Red Velvet Cake" to anyone who would take it. She gave out hundreds of them … for free! Because of this story, Red Velvet Cake earned the nicknames "Waldorf-Astoria Cake" and "$100 cake!"

Meanwhile, in Austin, TX in the 1930s, Mr. John A. Adams started getting very rich selling vanilla and food dyes because of the cake's growing popularity. He and his wife, Betty, ate the Red Velvet Cake at the Waldorf-Astoria hotel and then got the recipe from the woman who was handing it out on buses! John and Betty began printing and selling the recipe on cake boxes, next to their bottled vanilla and red food dye all over the US!

The featured ingredient: Beets!

★ **Beets are a member of an order of flowering plants that includes cacti,** amaranth, carnations, quinoa, spinach, and even Venus fly traps!

★ **Modern beets derived from wild sea beets that originated around the coasts of the Middle East, Africa, and Europe.** Ancient varieties of beets were white and black in color rather than red!

★ **Beet juice has been used as a natural red dye for hundreds of years.** The Victorians used beets to dye their hair red.

★ **To clean stained fingers (also known as "pink fingers") from cooking beets, rub with lemon juice and salt** before washing with soap and water.

★ **Beets contain many vitamins and minerals** such as vitamin C, potassium, iron, and manganese. Regular beets contain no more than 10% sugar, while sugar beets contain 20% sugar.

red velvet doughnut holes

ingredients

1½ C all-purpose flour

3 T unsweetened cocoa powder

1½ tsp baking powder

½ tsp baking soda

1 tsp cinnamon

3 T chocolate chips

pinch salt

2 eggs

½ C white sugar

1 C milk

1 tsp vanilla extract

2½ T white vinegar

2 T salted butter, softened

1 C cooked or canned beets (NOT pickled beets!)

oil (for cooking)

preheat+measure+whisk

Preheat your oven to 400 degrees F. Have your kids measure your dry ingredients into a large bowl: **1½ cups of flour, 3 tablespoons of unsweetened cocoa powder, 1½ teaspoons of baking powder, ½ teaspoon of baking soda, 1 teaspoon of cinnamon, 3 tablespoons of chocolate chips,** and **a pinch of salt.** Whisk to combine.

crack+mix

Have your kids crack **2 eggs** and combine with ½ **cup of white sugar, 1 cup of milk, 1 teaspoon of vanilla, 2½ tablespoons of vinegar, and 2 tablespoons of softened butter** in a separate large bowl. Blend with a hand blender or mixer until smooth. Add **1 cup of cooked or canned beets** and blend again until smooth.

well+add

Make a well in the center of your dry ingredients and have your kids slowly whisk in the wet ingredients. Add a little more milk if the batter appears to be too thick.

pour+pop+turn

Put about ¼ **tablespoon of oil** in the bottom of each well in a mini-muffin pan and heat the empty pan until hot. Carefully pour in about 1 tablespoon of the batter into each cup. Pop them into the oven and bake for about 6 to 8 minutes. As soon as they get bubbly and brown around the edges, pull the muffin pan out of the oven and turn the doughnut holes quickly and carefully (a chopstick works great!). Continue baking for 3 to 4 more minutes until cooked though. Remove and cool. Roll in *Mint Dust* (see recipe below) and enjoy!

- -

mint dust

ingredients

¼ to ½ C sugar   1 to 2 fresh mint leaves

measure+massage

Measure ¼ **to ½ cup of suga**r into a small bowl and add **1 to 2 mint leaves.** Have your kids massage the mint leaves into the sugar, allowing the mint oils and flavor to infuse into the sugar. You can let the mint rest in the sugar for 5 to 10 minutes and even up to one week!

- -

red velvet shakes

ingredients

3 C milk   1 small cooked or canned beet
3 T unsweetened cocoa powder   handful of chocolate chips
5 T sugar/honey/agave   2 C ice

combine+blend

Have kids measure and combine in a blender or large pitcher for use with an immersion blender:
3 cups of milk, 3 tablespoons of cocoa powder, 5 tablespoons of sugar/honey/agave,
1 beet, and **a handful of chocolate chips.** Blend until smooth. Add **2 cups of ice** and blend again. Taste — does it need more cocoa, milk, sweetener? Adjust and enjoy!

(Almost) Hands-free Butternut Squash Risotto + Best Butternut Salad + Apricoty Squashy Sorbetti

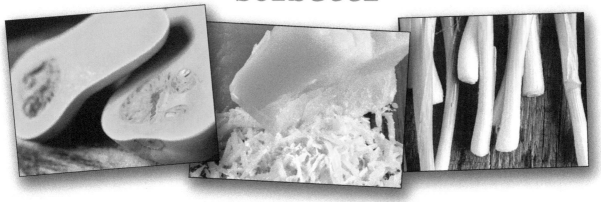

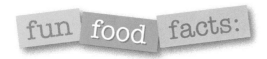

What is Risotto?

Risotto (rizz-OH-toe) is a famous rice dish from northern Italy cooked in broth until a creamy consistency is met. The broth may be meat, fish, or vegetable based. Many types of risotto contain butter, wine, and onion. It is one of the most common ways of cooking rice in Italy. In the Middle Ages, the Arabs first introduced rice to Italy and Spain, and people soon discovered the humid Mediterranean climate was perfect for growing short-grain varieties of rice. As the popularity of rice grew in Italy, so did the profits made from those selling it. **Milan is most known for its relationship with rice and risotto.** Slow-cooking local rice and adding rich spices like saffron helped Milan create the now-famous dish, *Risotto alla Milanese*.

The featured ingredient: Butternut Squash!

★ **Though squash has been around for over 10,000 years, the butternut variety didn't exist until the 1940s.** The man who developed the butternut squash, Charles A. Leggett, was neither a farmer nor a scientist. When Leggett moved to a farm in Massachusetts to spend more time outdoors, he never wanted to grow crops. However, he hated to see his land "lying idle." He wanted a squash for his family to eat that was tasty, compact, and easy to grow and prepare. He started crossing the gooseneck squash with other varieties. Leggett loved the squash that he created so much that he started to brag to everyone that it was "as smooth as butter and sweet as a nut" — thus, butternut squash was born!

- ★ **Butternut squash is a great source of vitamin A** with one serving providing 213% of your daily vitamin A requirement.

- ★ **Butternut squash seeds are similar to pumpkin seeds in the fact that they can be eaten for a nutritious snack.**

- ★ **Native American tribes grew over 40 types of squash**. They boiled or roasted it and preserved the flesh in syrup. At first, European settlers were not impressed by squash, that is, until they had to survive through the cold winter. Pumpkins and squash then became staples in their diet.

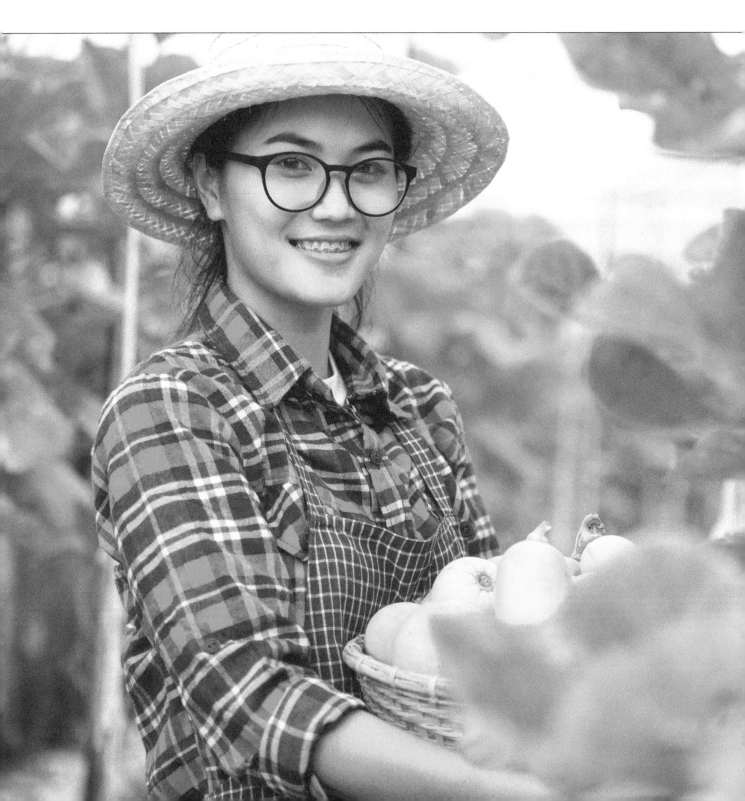

(almost) hands-free butternut squash risotto

ingredients

2 stalks green onions
2 garlic cloves
3 T butter
2 T olive oil
2 C instant brown rice
14 oz vegetable broth
½ C milk

1 C fresh, cooked (or frozen + thawed) butternut squash
½ tsp white wine vinegar
salt and pepper
½ C grated Parmesan cheese (+ more for sprinkling)
½ tsp apple cider (or white) vinegar

thaw/pre-cook

If using frozen butternut squash, thaw according to package directions. If using fresh butternut squash, cook either by steam-baking, roasting, boiling, microwaving, or baking.

To steam-bake: Cut the squash in half, lengthwise and place cut side down into a 9x13" glass baking dish. Add ½ cup water to the baking dish and cover tightly with foil. Bake at 350 degrees F for 1 hour. Remove from oven and let cool slightly before handling. Flip the squash over and scoop out the seeds and membranes and discard.

To roast: Slice the butternut squash into ½-inch thick half-moon slices, or peel and dice the squash (removing seeds and membranes). Toss it with some olive oil and roast at 400 degrees F for 35 to 40 minutes.

To boil: Peel the squash, slice in half lengthwise, and remove the seeds and membranes. Dice the flesh and boil for 15 to 20 minutes, or until soft.

To microwave: Cut several slits into the flesh to allow steam to escape as it cooks through. For a medium-sized squash, cook for about 10 minutes in the microwave. Remove carefully, as it will be very hot. Let cool before handling.

To bake: Cut the butternut squash in half lengthwise, scoop out seeds and membranes, and place flesh-side down on a foil-lined baking sheet. Bake at 350 degrees F for 50 to 55 minutes. Remove from oven and let cool before handling.

chop+brown

Have your kids chop up **1 cup of butternut squash**. Add some oil to a skillet on your stovetop and brown the squash until soft. (If you are also making the *Best Butternut Salad*, brown an additional ½ **to 1 cup of butternut squash** for this recipe and set to the side.)

mince+melt

Have your kids mince **2 stalks green onion** and **2 garlic cloves** into little bits. Add **3 tablespoons of butter** and **2 tablespoons of olive oil** to a skillet on your stovetop and heat over medium heat until butter is melted. Add the onion and garlic and cook for about 2 to 3 minutes, but don't brown! Turn off the heat on your skillet.

measure+stir

Have your kids measure and add **2 cups uncooked instant brown rice** to the skillet and stir to coat with the butter/oil. Then add **14 oz (1¾ cups) of vegetable broth, ½ cup of milk,** and **1 cup of your chopped butternut squash**.

simmer+mix

Turn your heat back on to medium and bring rice to a boil. Then reduce heat to low and simmer for 5 minutes until the rice is tender. Mix in **½ cup of grated cheese** and **salt and pepper** to taste. Stir in **½ teaspoon of vinegar** to finish and top each serving with an extra sprinkle of Parmesan cheese!

• •

best butternut salad

ingredients

1 stalk green onion	1 T white vinegar
1 fresh apricot (or 2 dried)	¼ C pre-cooked and browned butternut
3 T olive oil	squash
1 T honey or sugar	2 C spinach/lettuce/arugula
¼ T salt	¼ C grated Parmesan cheese
pinch black pepper	

chop+measure+blend

Have your kids chop up **1 green onion stalk** and **1 fresh apricot** (or 2 dried). Add to a food processor, your blender, or big bowl to use with your immersion blender. Then have your kids measure and add to the bowl/blender: **3 tablespoons of olive oil, 1 tablespoon of honey or sugar, ¼ tablespoon of salt, a pinch of black pepper,** and **1 tablespoon of vinegar.** Blend the dressing until creamy and thick.

add+toss

Pour dressing into a bowl and add **½ to 1 cup of pre-cooked and browned butternut squash** and **2 cups fresh spinach/lettuce/arugula.** Toss the salad with the dressing, sprinkle ¼ **cup grated cheese** on top and enjoy immediately!

apricoty squashy sorbetti

ingredients

3 fresh apricots (or 6 dried)
½ C honey or sugar

¼ C fresh, cooked (or frozen + thawed)
butternut squash
4 C ice

cut+add+blend

Have your kids cut up **3 fresh apricots** (or 6 dried) into quarters or smaller and throw into a blender or bowl for use with an immersion blender — peels and all! Add ½ **cup of honey or sugar,** ¼ **cup of cooked butternut squash** and **4 cups of ice.** Blend everything until super smooth and thick. Taste — does it need more sugar? Adjust, serve, and enjoy!

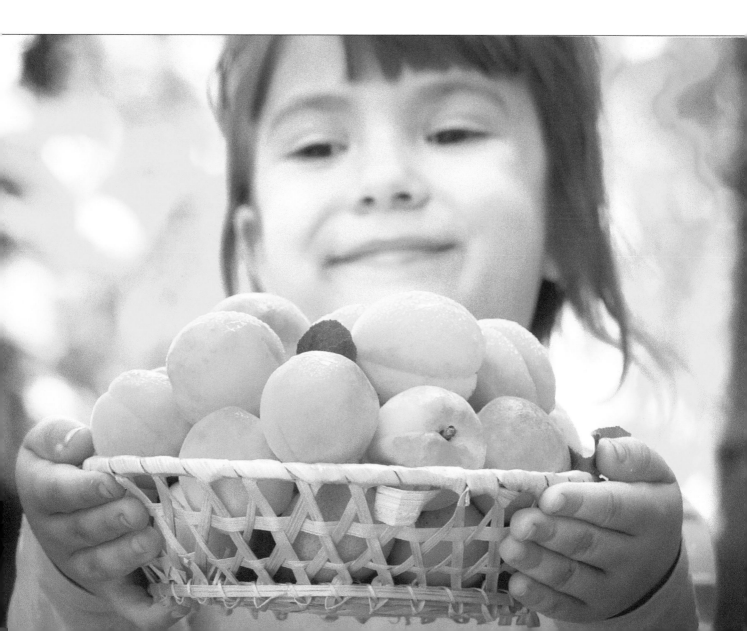

German Apple-Oat Streusel Pancakes
+ Cinnamon Apple Streusel Smoothies

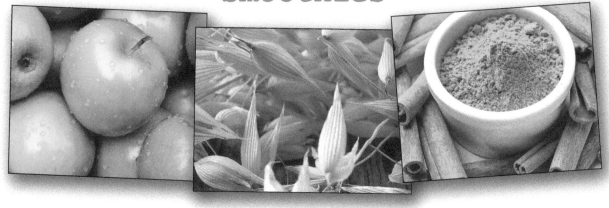

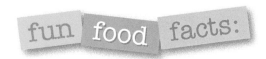

What is streusel?

Streusel (STREW-sill) is a German word meaning "something scattered or sprinkled."
Traditionally, it is a sweet crumb topping consisting of sugar, butter, and flour, mixed at a 1:1: 2 ratio. Streuselkuchen, or crumb cake, is a light, moist, yeasted dessert adorned with a sweet, buttery crumb topping. While it is believed that streusel originated in Silesia, a former Prussian province near modern-day Poland, it is most often associated with German cuisine.

As of the early 21st century, the cake continues to be enjoyed in Germany as a dessert or an accompaniment to coffee. It is also a familiar treat in other world regions that claim large populations of people of German descent, such as the Midwestern states in the US and parts of South America.

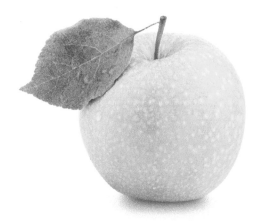

The featured ingredient: Apples!

★ **The Granny Smith apple was named for Maria Ann Smith** who created it from a hybrid seedling in Australia in the 1800s.

★ **Apples come in all shades of red, green, and yellow.**

★ **Apples are grown throughout the US in all 50 states.** Apple trees take approximately 4-5 years to yield their first fruit and can grow as tall as 40 feet. They can even live over 100 years!

★ **Apples are a great source of the fiber pectin.** One apple has five grams of fiber.

★ **The apple tree originated in an area between the Caspian and the Black Sea,** and apples were a favorite fruit of the ancient Greeks and Romans.

★ **Apples are a member of the rose family.**

★ **25% of an apple's volume is air.** That is why they float!

german apple-oat streusel pancakes

ingredients

1 large Granny Smith apple
2 eggs
1½ C + ⅓ C all-purpose flour
1½ tsp baking powder
1 C milk
2 tsp vanilla extract

½ tsp cinnamon
¼ C unsalted butter, cold
½ C brown sugar
⅓ C oats
honey, agave, or maple syrup for drizzling on pancakes

pronounce+chop

Start the recipe by pronouncing *streusel* together 3 times fast (STREW-sill)! Have your kids grate or chop up **1 Granny Smith apple** into VERY fine bits, or carefully shred with a grater, and set to the side.

crack+beat+measure

Start to prepare the batter by having kids crack and beat **2 eggs** in a large bowl. Then measure and combine **1½ cups of flour** and **1½ teaspoons of baking powder** in a large bowl. Add the beaten eggs with **1 cup of milk, 2 teaspoons of vanilla extract,** and **¼ teaspoon of cinnamon**. Whisk until smooth. Then stir in shredded or chopped apple.

blend+crumb+toast

Streusel time! Have kids combine ¼ **cup of cold butter,** ⅓ **cup of flour,** ½ **cup of brown sugar,** ⅓ **cup of oats,** and ¼ teaspoon cinnamon into a bowl and blend with a fork or clean fingers until you have coarse crumbs. Reserve ¼ cup of the raw streusel topping to add to your pancakes later on. Toast the remaining streusel topping by itself in your non-stick skillet for 3 to 6 minutes on low heat, stirring with a wooden spoon. Remove the toasted streusel from your skillet and set to the side.

sprinkle+flip

Pancake time! Heat your skillet over medium heat. For mini-pancakes, ladle 2 to 4 tablespoons of batter onto your skillet and cook for 1 minute before sprinkling the batter with the un-toasted streusel. Cook pancakes 2 to 3 minutes on the first side (until golden brown) and then flip and cook another 2 to 3 minutes on the second side. The streusel will start to cook into the top of the pancake so it shouldn't fall off during the flip. Divide the un-toasted streusel evenly among the pancakes.

eat+exclaim

Spoon the reserved toasted streusel onto the top of the pancakes. Serve warm with **maple syrup, honey, agave, or other syrup** of your choice and eat immediately. Don't forget to exclaim, "That was delicious!" in German—*Das war köstlich!* (dahs var kust-leekh).

- -

cinnamon apple streusel smoothies

ingredients

1 Granny Smith apple	3 T honey or sugar (or 1½ tsp stevia)
2 medium bananas	½ tsp vanilla extract
2 C milk	dash cinnamon
2 T oats	1 C ice

chop+dash+blend

Have kids chop up **1 Granny Smith apple** and **2 bananas** and add to your blender. Measure **2 cups of milk, 2 tablespoons of oats, 3 tablespoons of honey or sugar (or 1½ teaspoons of stevia), ½ teaspoon of vanilla extract, dash of cinnamon,** and **1 cup of ice** and add into the blender on top of the fruit. Blend until smooth and creamy. Drink and enjoy!

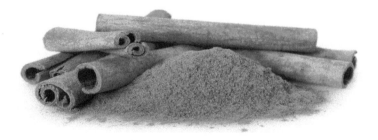

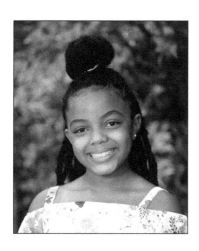

Congratulations to Young Chef Saniyah!
The Farm to Table Cover Star

How did you first get interested in cooking?

Response: I first got interested in cooking because I watched my family cook delicious food.

Your cookbook cover photo was taken during an online Sticky Fingers Cooking class where students made the Chef's Choice Magical One-Pot Pasta + Enchanting Green Goddess Salad + Frosty Fruit Sorbet Blender Wizardry recipe. What did you enjoy about that particular recipe?

Response: I really enjoyed the sorbet because of how fun it was, but also found it interesting that you could put almost anything in the pasta.

What does the phrase "farm to table" mean to you and your family?

Response: "Farm to table" to us means that someone sells us fruit and vegetables fresh from a farm and then we cook it to put it on the table.

What is one of your favorite ingredients to cook with and why?

Response: One of my favorite ingredients to cook with is eggs because you can make many things with them.

Why do you think it's important for kids to get involved in the kitchen?

Response: I think it's important for kids to get involved because when they grow up, they have to cook for themselves.

What advice would you give to young or aspiring chefs?

Response: Don't give up if you make a mistake. Even professionals mess up. It may be hard to do something, but keep trying.

If you could have any cooking superpower, what would it be and why?

Response: I would have the ability to cook super fast because a lot of times I don't have time to cook.

What's a favorite food pun or joke of yours? No joke can be too cheesy for us ;)

Response: What did the spagetti say to the meatball? Ans: You know I don't like meat on me right?

VERY GRATEFUL ACKNOWLEGMENTS

"We are each other's harvest; we are each other's business; we are each other's magnitude and bond." - Gwendolyn Brooks

Thank you to all of our Sticky Fingers Cooking students. Always enthusiastic and willing to try new foods. We couldn't have made this book without your feedback. Keep questioning, learning, and thriving. Remember that those who cook well are never without friends—you just need a longer table.

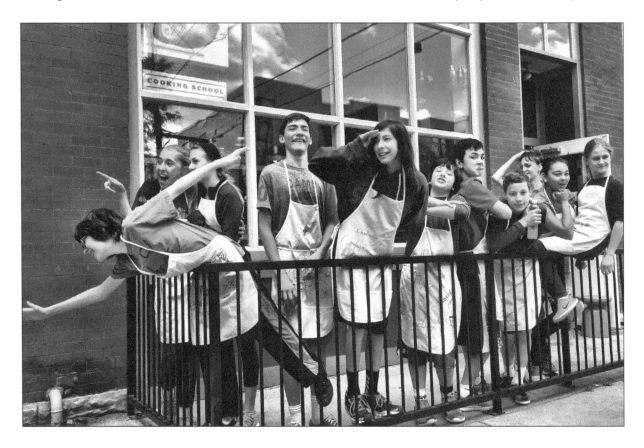

A massive thank you to our exceptional team of Chef Instructors who are the heart and soul of Sticky Fingers Cooking. We flourish because of your talents and zest for teaching. You gently plant and grow the delights of cooking and healthy eating into your students every day. We love and so appreciate that we've been able to include so many of your awesome photos of the students cooking in your amazingly fun and delicious classes.

Gratitude given to Saniyah, and her family, for submitting her gorgeously vibrant photo for our cover. My most sincere acknowledgements to Amy & Peregrin Marshall of Web501, Sarah Morrissey of Juniper Accounting, and Bart Writer and Randy Williams of Madison Financial who's continued support help consciously grow Sticky Fingers Cooking. To Jennifer Gauerke of YellowDog Denver, to Shannon McLaughlin, Susan English, and the numerous photographers (including my daughter, Ava Fletter) who each contributed to this deliciously lush book.

I'm profoundly thankful and in awe of our Sticky Fingers Cooking administrative team, Joe Hall, Katie Brennan, Kimberly Douglas, Lucy Warenski, Amanda Adams, Lauren Frontiera, Maggie Whittum, Chloe Sundberg, Francine Huang, Kate Bezak, Jessi Cano, Robin Pearce, Alli Doyle, Eileen Leno, Dylan Sabuco, Jacy Shoener, Caroline Duffy, and Amy Carter. Your united combination of enthusiasm, compassion, creativity, grit, wit, and steadfast attention sow and harvest the seeds of success every day.

A good editor can be handed a bundle of recipes, thoughts, ideas, and words and make them flow together harmoniously. Precisely what Emily Moore from Red Pen LLC and her daughter Piper Sturgis, whose expertise and eagle-eyed focus on details, deliver. I'm forever grateful.

Thank you to the divine Francine Huang. She helped to carefully cultivate and format the recipes we choose for this book, a challenge considering we have over 800 recipes to consider.

I was fortunate enough to co-write some of the recipes in this book with the abundantly talented Jacqui Gabel. She is a joy and a deliciously brilliant friend.

Thank you to the multi-talented Kate Bezak for her skillful wordsmithing. Kate cultivated wonderful activities and wrote many of the resources found in this book. Kate's thoughtfulness, creativity, and intelligence make her a complete joy to work with.

A million and one thanks to the massively creative Natasha McCone, who is our book layout artist. Her positive energy is evergreen, and she is an invaluable member of our cookbook team.

My beloved mom, Laura Hall, planted the power in me to believe in myself and pursue my dreams. I cannot imagine my life without her eternal love and the endless faith she always seems to have in me.

This cookbook was exquisitely designed, in its entirety, by the mind-blowingly visionary, multi-talented and ever-fascinating, Joe Hall. His optimism knows no bounds. Joe is a friend and an inspiration to so many people. To my good fortune, he is also my Dad. This book is dedicated to him.

I am forever grateful for my precious children, Ava, Liliana, and Vivian. I am incredibly proud of them. My deepest roots of love proliferate, intertwine, and expand for them every day. Beyond measure. Beyond compare.

To thank my magnificent husband, Ryan Fletter, would not be enough. He is a loving father, a fantastic restaurateur, a perfect partner, and so much more—continuous appreciation to Ryan for loving and growing with me for over 25 years. And counting.

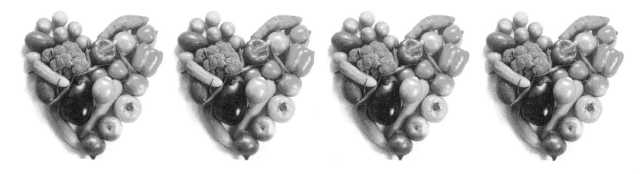

THE HANDY INDEX

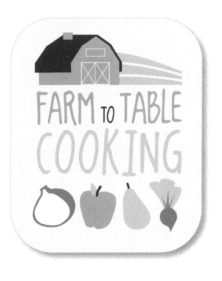

About the Author

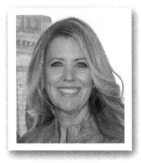

Erin Fletter

FOOD GEEK-IN-CHIEF

Erin Fletter is passionate about getting kids to not just eat, but actually crave healthy food. Erin's three enthusiastic daughters are her first round of recipe taste testers and she is never reluctant to push their culinary boundaries.

Erin loves creating hands on recipes for children that bring together fresh ingredients, global flavors, math, geography, language, nutrition, food history—and a big dash of tasty fun. Erin also writes terrible jokes about food that make everyone groan.

Erin has an extensive background in the food and wine industry and used that experience to start Sticky Fingers Cooking, a mobile and online cooking school. Sticky Fingers Cooking now has hundreds of cooking classes each week in multiple cities and has taught over 50,000 kids how to cook. Erin lives in Denver, Colorado, with her husband, three daughters, two cats and one dog; all of whom are extremely well fed.

"Wow, Chef Erin! You really write ALL of these recipes for Sticky Fingers? Good thing your food is a million times better than your jokes."

- Avery, age 6

Cookbook Freebies and more!
Open Up a New World of so many
COOL'inary Possibilities

CPSIA information can be obtained
at www.ICGtesting.com
Printed in the USA
LVHW070843240322
714288LV00009B/123